MANAGEMENT OF TYPE 2
DIABETES MELLITUS

A PRACTICAL GUIDE

Commissioning Editor: Alison Taylor
Project Development Manager: Kim Benson
Project Manager: Elouise Ball
Designer: Charles Gray
Illustration Manager: Merlyn Harvey
Illustrator: Richard Morris

MANAGEMENT OF TYPE 2

DIABETES MELLITUS

A PRACTICAL GUIDE

Second edition

Steven Levene MA, MB, BChir, FRCGP
General Practitioner,
East Leicester Medical Practice
Leicester, UK

And

Richard Donnelly MD, PhD, FRCP, FRACP
Professor and Associate Dean
(Graduate-Entry Medicine),
University of Nottingham, Nottingham, UK

Foreword by *Professor Richard Hobbs*
Head of Department of Primary Care & General
Practice, University of Birmingham, UK

ELSEVIER
BUTTERWORTH
HEINEMANN

EDINBURGH LONDON NEW YORK OXFORD
PHILADELPHIA ST LOUIS SYDNEY TORONTO 2008

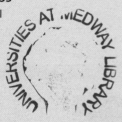

BUTTERWORTH
HEINEMANN
ELSEVIER

© 2008, Elsevier Limited

No part of this publication may be reproduced, stored in a retrieval system, or transmitted in any form or by any means, electronic, mechanical, photocopying, recording or otherwise, without the prior permission of the Publishers. Permissions may be sought directly from Elsevier's Health Sciences Rights Department, 1600 John F. Kennedy Boulevard, Suite 1800, Philadelphia, PA 19103-2899, USA: phone: (+1) 215 239 3804; fax: (+1) 215 239 3805; or, e-mail: healthpermissions@elsevier.com. You may also complete your request on-line via the Elsevier homepage (http://www.elsevier.com), by selecting 'Support and contact' and then 'Copyright and Permission'.

First edition 2003

ISBN: 978 0 08 0449838

British Library Cataloguing in Publication Data
A catalogue record for this book is available from the British Library
Library of Congress Cataloging in Publication Data
A catalog record for this book is available from the Library of Congress

Note
Knowledge and best practice in this field are constantly changing. As new research and experience broaden our knowledge, changes in practice, treatment and drug therapy may become necessary or appropriate. Readers are advised to check the most current information provided (i) on procedures featured or (ii) by the manufacturer of each product to be administered, to verify the recommended dose or formula, the method and duration of administration, and contraindications. It is the responsibility of the practitioner, relying on their own experience and knowledge of the patient, to make diagnoses, to determine dosages and the best treatment for each individual patient, and to take all appropriate safety precautions. To the fullest extent of the law, neither the Publisher nor the Authors assume any liability for any injury and/or damage to persons or property arising out of or related to any use of the material contained in this book.

The Publisher

Printed in China

CONTENTS

Dr Steven Levene MA, MB, BChir, FRCGP
Principal in General Practice, East Leicester Medical Practice, Leicester

Dr Levene trained at Cambridge University and St Mary's Hospital Medical School, London and ha en a full-time partner in a busy Leicester inner-city practice since 1986. He is also a trainer and audit assessor with the Leicestershire Northamptonshire Rutland Vocational Training Scheme. His interests are in diabetes mellitus, ophthalmology, research, consultation skills (a particular interest) and pain management (including acupuncture). During a sabbatical in 2004 he worked in the Pain Management Service, University Hospitals of Leicester NHS Trust.

Dr Levene has written two books on diabetes and published two peer-reviewed papers: the first on the characteristics of psychiatric inpatients and the second on the prevalence of microalbuminuria in diabetics in the community.

Professor Richard Donnelly MD, PhD, FRCP, FRACP
Professor of Vascular Medicine & Associate Dean, Faculty of Medicine & Health Sciences, University of Nottingham & Derby Hospitals NHS Foundation Trust

Professor Donnelly has been a Professor of Vascular Medicine in the University of Nottingham since 1997, is an Honorary Consultant Physician (Diabetes/Medicine) and Director of NHS Research & Development in Derby Hospitals NHS Foundation Trust, and is an Associate Dean for the University of Nottingham Graduate-Entry Medical programme based in Derby (this is an innovative, fast-track 4-year medical course). He has clinical and research interests in the vascular complications of diabetes (including detection, mechanisms and pharmacological intervention), insulin resistance and the evidenced-based use of disease-modifying drugs to improve symptoms and survival in high-risk patients with diabetes. His career to date has included a 2-year (1992–1994) British Heart Foundation Fellowship at Stanford University, California, working with Dr Gerald Reaven (famous for describing the insulin resistance syndrome in his 1988 ADA Banting Lecture), and, from 1994 to 1997, the position of Senior Lecturer & Consultant Physician in the Diabetes Centre, Royal Prince Alfred Hospital, University of Sydney, Australia.

Professor Donnelly is Editor-in-chief of *Diabetes, Obesity & Metabolism*, an international Medline-listed journal that focuses on clinical and experimental pharmacology in this area (impact factor 2.1), and he is an Executive Editor (Diabetes & Endocrinology) of the *British Journal of Clinical Pharmacology*. He has published over 160 peer-reviewed papers on aspects of diabetes and cardiovascular disease.

The management of diabetes mellitus has become mainstream medicine. The reasons for this are self-evident considering the rapid rise in prevalence of type 2 diabetes in all developing and developed economies. As the data in chapter one illustrates, this translates to high proportions of the population suffering the disease, with at least 2% identified but probably nearer 4.5% of the population at risk in England. The latter figure would encompass 2.4 million. As Levene and Donnelly point out, there are many factors that will drive these figures even higher, most notably increasingly sedentary lifestyles associated with increased rates of obesity. So, one very important factor that has driven diabetes mainstream has been that it is such a common chronic disorder facing health services. The increased detection of diabetes, that increased numbers of people who need active management and secondary preventive strategies, and diabetes care has increasingly become an activity that can only be delivered systematically within primary care. There has therefore been a sea change in health provision in the United Kingdom during the past decade, that has seen virtually all the management of type 2 diabetes move from hospital to community settings. What this shift of care necessitates is better access to educational materials on diabetes for the generalist, whether in the community or hospital practice. This is the rationale for this new book on managing type 2 diabetes, and very welcome it is too.

Levene and Donnelly have managed to write a new text book that will act as a reference point and a practical guide to the generalist. The authors have succeeded in producing an unusually up-to-date text book (which is at least partly a measure of the much shorter lead times possible now in modern publishing). Indeed, the chapters importantly indicate where forthcoming studies or reviews are likely to add to the evidence base in the coming year or two, providing a useful 'heads up' to the reader. So the evidence base is contemporary and the authors have, wherever possible, based their recommendations on the major consensus guidelines that have been incorporated into the National Service Framework for Diabetes, the NICE publications relating to diabetes, and Cochrane Reviews. However, the authors have added another essential ingredient to this authoritative and contemporary feel, namely accessibility. The book is laid out and written in a style that makes for easy overall reading, but also easy access if particular snippets of information are required, such as how to initiate insulin in chapter three or details on the current regulations around driving (chapter six).

The chapters are laid out logically. Importantly, there is a full chapter available on lifestyle with important recommendations around exercise and smoking cessation as well as dietary control. Where possible, the authors have provided options and produced a practical flavour of how behavioural interventions might work within a primary care setting, quoting a number of the theoretical models that exist for improving the likely better patient concordance with lifestyle advice. The chapter on glycaemiac control is comprehensive across all types of therapy, including insulin use, and it also provides information on the newest class of drugs, (the GLP1 analogues and DPP4 inhibitors) which have only gained licensed approvals this year. The chapter on reducing cardiovascular risk provides useful recommendations around treating the common vascular risk factors that co-exist in diabetes as well as summarising the evidence base for preventive strategies. This is a large chapter, which reflects the greater recognition of the vascular risk associated with diabetes mellitus – it is essentially a disease of accelerated cardiovascular risk associated with raised glycaemia.

The chapter on diabetes complications includes the upgraded recommendations around fundoscopy screening, in addition to useful information on the under-recognised and under-managed problem of erectile dysfunction. The 'living with diabetes' chapter is particularly comprehensive with useful information on standard areas such as driving, employment and travel, supplemented by novel sections around the cultural aspects of multi-ethnic societies such as the UK which may manifest on better management of diabetes. The importance of team work and careful planning of diabetes care in any modern health system is exemplified by a whole chapter devoted to the organisation and delivery of optimal diabetes care. This section includes recommendations around the structure of clinics, frequency of reviews and has a section of audit as well. The book ends with a number of useful appendices including a complete drug formulary for diabetes, summaries of the National Service Frameworks standards and Quality and Outcome Framework indicators that relate to diabetes; and an extensive section on resources, including useful websites from around the world.

So, in summary, this book is very much aimed at the primary care physician in any organised health system where much of diabetes care occurs in the community. As the authors state themselves, the text book should be essential reading for any GP with a special interest in diabetes, but I would wholeheartedly recommend it for a much wider readership to any generalist whether in primary or secondary care setting, whether medical or housing, whether in training or established practice. The authors have achieved an impressive new text book for the modern management of diabetes mellitus and it deserves to be read cover to cover.

Professor Richard Hobbs

The management of type 2 diabetes mellitus and its complications accounts for an increasing proportion of primary care's workload. Both those who use (patients) and those who fund (taxpayers via government) the service now expect practices to deliver appropriate and effective care universally to a high standard, and "fit for purpose".

Professionals face a continuous and enormous flow of new research findings, new guidelines from various learned bodies and new information about treatments. Before updating their practice, non-specialists who deliver diabetes care need to evaluate carefully all this new information, with a shrewd awareness of any potential clinical, organisational and financial pitfalls. The gap between the targets that the expert bodies advise and/or managers expect and that which a stretched primary care service can deliver for each individual patient in reality may not be always bridgeable.

We have written this book for the whole primary health-care team, concentrating throughout on providing practical up-to-date advice to enable clinicians, with their patients, to make optimal appropriate choices. We believe that many of the concepts discussed here (e.g. improving vascular risk factors, enabling self-management, consulting effectively and using psychological techniques to influence health-related behaviour) are relevant to most patient–professional encounters, even when the problem is not diabetes mellitus.

Since one of our main aims is to provide guidance for practices to achieve maximum points in the QOF indicators of the GP contract, the text has references to relevant sections of both the QOF and the NSF. This book also covers the relevant aspects of diabetes in Curriculum Statement 15.6 recently prepared by the Royal College of General Practitioners, which forms the basis of the new membership examination and the competencies expected of General Practitioners. When the singular is found in the text and applies to both genders, the convention of masculine terms he, his or him have been used, to avoid the unwieldy "he or she", "his or her", and "him or her".

For the second edition, we have re-organised, expanded and re-written most of the text. Hopefully, readers will find something useful from the following pages.

Steven Levene,
Richard Donnelly

Steven Levene wishes to thank the following professional colleagues for allowing him to "pick their brains": George Alberti, Richard Baker, Mary Burden, Tim Coleman, Melanie Davies, Michael Drucquer, Azhar Farooqi, David Kingdon, Ian Lawrence, Steve Longworth, Paul McNally, Sue Moriarty and Tim Terry.

The final responsibility for what follows is the authors'.

SETTING THE SCENE

WHY IS PRIMARY CARE IMPORTANT IN THE MANAGEMENT OF TYPE 2 DIABETES PATIENTS?

Diabetes mellitus is categorised as a metabolic disease, characterised by chronic hyperglycaemia. The subgroup, type 2, accounts for a substantial majority of patients with diabetes. In primary care, diabetics can present with a wide range of problems, either as a direct manifestation of diabetes or with diabetes being a significant contributor to the presentation.

Although secondary care can deliver high-quality care to individual patients with diabetes, there are compelling reasons why primary care should take a greater, or even leading, role in the delivery of care to patients with diabetes, leaving secondary care to concentrate on patients with more complex and challenging problems. These reasons include:

- the significantly greater morbidity and mortality associated with diabetes
- the increasing prevalence of diabetes and demands upon the service
- the importance of quality in the delivery of care to patients with diabetes
- the suitability of primary care for managing many chronic diseases.

THE SIGNIFICANTLY GREATER MORBIDITY AND MORTALITY ASSOCIATED WITH DIABETES

Even GPs without a special interest in diabetes are likely to encounter patients with diabetes or associated problems in their routine surgeries. Diabetics, especially those with type 2, are prone to a wide and devastating range of complications, predominately vascular in origin. In 1998 the United Kingdom Prospective Diabetes Study (UKPDS) reported that, for many diabetes complications, the onset could be delayed or the effect reduced by appropriate interventions (UKPDS 1998a, b, c), many of which can be and are, ideally, provided by primary care. Compared with the general population, type 2 diabetics carry a markedly greater risk of suffering myocardial infarction and stroke, particularly if additional risk factors are present (as they often are).

Diabetes care needs to include evidence-based aggressive interventions that minimise cardiovascular risk (Byrne 2000), discussed in greater detail in Chapters 2 and 4, as well as optimal management of the disease itself, i.e. glycaemic control and disease-specific complications (discussed in greater detail in Chapters 3 and 5, respectively).

INCREASING PREVALENCE OF DIABETES AND DEMANDS UPON THE SERVICE

The prevalence of type 2 diabetes continues to increase, particularly in certain subgroups such as Indo-Asians, with a greater incidence of vascular disease in these already high-risk individuals. This rising prevalence will lead to a greater workload, with substantial and increasing financial consequences, not only for the NHS. Effective, sustained and coordinated strategies to prevent or delay the onset of diabetes need to be implemented to counter this rise in its prevalence.

Ideally, primary care should be responsible for most routine diabetes surveillance, while secondary care manages late-stage complications (e.g. myocardial infarction, stroke, dialysis and angioplasty) and introduces new technologies (e.g. insulin pumps).

IMPORTANCE OF QUALITY IN DELIVERING CARE TO PATIENTS WITH DIABETES

The serious consequences and increasing prevalence of diabetes mellitus have driven the continuous quest to develop effective care and deliver it to those affected by or at risk of developing this disease. Patients with chronic diseases do require and should receive ongoing suitable care, based upon the implementation of agreed and justified protocols in combination with audit to evaluate performance and guide future changes. It is appropriate that the on-going responsibility for delivering this care should be "owned" by whoever "manages" the patient.

Poor organisation risks minimising the benefit that diabetic patients can obtain from professionals' often-considerable knowledge and skills. Unfortunately, some diabetics do not have regular contact with their practices, and those who do attend can receive a variable standard of care (Audit Commission 2000).

Organising and monitoring the delivery of high-quality care is discussed in Chapter 7. Its importance has been recognised by government policy and supported by the publication of various authoritative guidelines. Implementing much of this guidance may sometimes require additional resources.

SUITABILITY OF PRIMARY CARE TO MANAGE CHRONIC DISEASES

In 2001 the National Service Framework (NSF) for Diabetes published a list of 12 "standards" (see Appendix 2 defining areas of care that will need to be delivered): these include prevention, diagnosis, empowerment, clinical care, emergencies, pregnancy and long-term complications. Eight of the NSF standards are relevant to the management of type 2 diabetes in primary care. (Text in this book specific to these standards will be accompanied by a box in the margin giving details of the relevant standard.)

Unlike acute diseases in which patients are often passive recipients of medical care, successful chronic-disease management requires the patient to be an active partner in the process (Holman 2000). This principle underpins "patient empowerment", cited in NSF Standard 3 (see Appendix 2). If patients are regarded as the main managers of their chronic disease, with the professionals acting as both guide and coach, then better outcomes are more likely. Primary care professionals are well placed to facilitate this, since:

- primary care is geared to focusing on the 'whole' patient and to addressing his agenda
- primary care is accessible
- patients usually prefer the continuity of seeing their GP and practice nurse rather than a succession of junior hospital doctors in a busy hospital diabetes clinic.

Although intensive blood-glucose control increases therapy costs (drugs, monitoring, clinic visits), the UKPDS argued that these are offset largely by significantly reduced costs of fewer complications, particularly those leading to hospital outpatient visits and/or admissions (Gray 2000).

Well-organised and highly motivated practices can provide both high-quality and cost-effective care for the majority of diabetics. Better management of chronic diseases can also provide health-care professionals with increased job satisfaction.

▶ KEY POINTS

- The main causes of morbidity and mortality in people with type 2 diabetes are cardiovascular.

- The core aims of the management of type 2 diabetes should include the reduction of cardiovascular risk, the improved well-being of patients, and greater patient autonomy.

- Collaboration between patients (achieving and maintaining an optimal lifestyle) and health-care professionals (implementing agreed evidence-based interventions) is more likely to achieve these aims.

- Patients own their disease, and thus they are at the centre of goal setting and disease management.

- Successful health education relies as much on modifying attitudes as on merely imparting information.

- The remorseless rise in the prevalence of type 2 diabetes will place increasing demands upon health services, especially primary care.

- Effective prevention strategies at all levels require immediate implementation with adequate resources to reduce the rising prevalence and impact of type 2 diabetes.

- Many of the interventions discussed in this book are relevant to more than one parameter or area.

WHAT IS TYPE 2 DIABETES MELLITUS?

OVERVIEW

DEFINITION OF DIABETES MELLITUS

Diabetes mellitus is a group of metabolic diseases characterised and diagnosed by a chronic elevation of blood glucose (hyperglycaemia) that results from defects in insulin secretion, insulin action or both. This may be accompanied by various disturbances of carbohydrate, protein and fat metabolism. The effect of different clinical manifestations may depend upon the underlying cause(s) of the diabetes, the degree of deficit of insulin action, coexisting conditions and the extent of diabetic tissue damage. Much of the morbidity and mortality in diabetics results from vascular damage.

CLASSIFICATION OF DIABETES MELLITUS

The World Health Organization's classification of diabetes (WHO 1985) has been adopted internationally. The American Diabetes Association re-examined the diagnostic criteria and classification and recommended modifications in 1997, subsequently agreed by WHO (The Expert Committee 1997, Alberti et al 1998). The terms type 1 and type 2 diabetes (Table 1.1) replaced the old categories of insulin-dependent diabetes mellitus (IDDM) and non-insulin-dependent diabetes mellitus (NIDDM). The older classification was based upon treatment (many NIDDM patients are on insulin), but did not indicate the nature of the underlying cause (Wroe 1997).

Types 1 and 2 diabetes are compared in Table 1.2.

TABLE 1.1 1997–1998 ADA and WHO classification of diabetes mellitus

Type 1

(beta-cell destruction, usually leading to absolute insulin deficiency)
Autoimmune
Idiopathic

Type 2

(may range from predominately insulin resistance with relative insulin deficiency to a predominately secretory defect with or without insulin resistance)

Other specific types

Genetic defects of beta-cell function
Genetic defects in insulin action

(cont'd)

TABLE 1.1 1997–1998 ADA and WHO classification of diabetes mellitus—Cont'd

Diseases of the exocrine pancreas

Endocrinopathies

Drug- or chemical-induced

Infections

Uncommon forms of immune-mediated diabetes

Other genetic syndromes sometimes associated with diabetes

Gestational diabetes mellitus (includes gestational impaired glucose tolerance)

TABLE 1.2 Comparison of the characteristics of types 1 and 2 diabetes mellitus (Beers 1999) © 2006 by Merck & Co., Inc., Whitehouse Station, NJ, USA

Characteristic	Type 1 diabetes	Type 2 diabetes
Commonest age at onset	Usually <30 years	Most often >30 years, but note recent trends
Associated obesity	No	Yes
Propensity to develop ketoacidosis (requiring insulin to prevent/control)	Yes	No
Presence of classic symptoms of hyperglycaemia at diagnosis	Yes, often severe	May be absent If present, often moderate
Endogenous insulin secretion	Very low to undetectable	Variable, but low relative to plasma glucose levels
Insulin resistance	Not present	Yes, but variable
Twin concurrence	<50%	>90%
Associated with specific HLA-D antigens	Yes	No
Islet cell antibodies at diagnosis	Yes	No
Islet pathology	Insulitis, selective loss of most beta cells	Smaller, normal-looking islets Amyloid deposits common
Associated increased risks for micro- and macrovascular disease	Yes	Yes
Hyperglycaemia responds to oral agents	No	Yes, initially in most patients

CRITERIA AND METHODS FOR THE DIAGNOSIS OF DIABETES MELLITUS

NSF ◀
2

CONCEPTS INVOLVED IN MAKING A DIAGNOSIS

Establishing a diagnosis of diabetes mellitus "should" be straightforward: the blood glucose level is either above or below the diagnostic threshold. However, consensus must be reached as to what level should be set as the diagnostic threshold (*criteria*) and which diagnostic test(s) to use (*methods*). Making the correct diagnosis reliably in an asymptomatic patient (half of type 2 patients at diagnosis) may pose a challenge.

CURRENT CRITERIA AND METHODS

The current recommendations are based on a 1998 WHO consultative document (Alberti et al 1998). The following criteria are for diagnosis *only*, and are *not* criteria for initiating treatment or therapeutic goals:

- Fasting (no caloric intake for at least 8 hours) plasma glucose level of 7.0 mmol/l (126 mg/dl) or greater

  or

- Random plasma glucose level of 11.1 mmol/l (200 mg/dl) or greater

  or

- 2 hour plasma glucose level (post 75 g glucose load) of 11.1 mmol/l or greater, from an oral glucose tolerance test (OGTT).

A *single* reading above the diagnostic threshold is sufficient to make the diagnosis if the patient has classic symptoms (e.g. thirst, polyuria, lethargy, blurred vision and weight loss); otherwise, if the patient is asymptomatic, diagnosis requires *two abnormal results on separate days*.

Although the OGTT is the "gold standard", it may be impractical as a first-line investigation in general practice, being undertaken when the fasting or random plasma glucose results fail to resolve diagnostic uncertainty, especially in patients whose fasting levels fall into the "impaired fasting glucose" range (see below), and who are thought to be at high risk of developing either diabetes or vascular disease.

Glycosuria, abnormal finger-prick blood glucose or elevated glycated haemoglobin suggest, but do not satisfy, the diagnostic criteria for diabetes.

RATIONALE FOR DIAGNOSTIC CRITERIA AND METHODS

The distribution of plasma glucose concentrations is a continuum; so there needs to be a threshold that separates those who are at a substantially increased risk of developing adverse outcomes caused by diabetes from those who are not (The Expert Committee 2003b). The medical, social and economic costs of making a diagnosis in those not at increased risk must be balanced against the costs of failing to diagnose those at increased risk.

Historically, this threshold was determined by the relationship between blood glucose levels and *micro*vascular complications in type 1 diabetics: however, it may be more important that this threshold is determined by the relationship between blood glucose levels and *macro*vascular risk in a wider population (i.e. those with either impaired glucose tolerance or type 2 diabetes).

The WHO and other bodies have adopted the ADA's diagnostic criteria (The Expert Committee 1997), but there have been different recommended optimal methods of diagnosis. The WHO prefers the OGTT, supported by evidence that 2 hour post-load plasma glucose levels were more accurate than fasting plasma glucose levels in identifying those at increased risk of death associated with hyperglycaemia (DECODE 1999). The drawback of ADA's preference for fasting plasma glucose levels is that "normal" results carry the risk of missing some diabetics, especially among the elderly and in some ethnic groups: the earliest defect in the natural history of beta cell dysfunction is the reduction of first-phase insulin release, associated with 2 hour post-load hyperglycaemia.

Although diabetes is "arbitrarily" and solely diagnosed on the basis of blood glucose levels, it should be regarded as a syndrome that includes other metabolic and haemodynamic features.

ORAL GLUCOSE TOLERANCE TEST (OGTT)

Standard protocol

After 3 or more days with a daily carbohydrate intake of at least 150 g, the OGTT should be performed in the morning after an overnight fast of 8–14 hours (during which plain water may be drunk). A venous blood sample is taken then a drink containing the equivalent of 75 g of glucose (e.g. Lucozade 388 ml) is consumed within 5 minutes. The subject should be seated, not smoke and take no unusual exercise during the test period. A second venous blood sample is taken exactly 2 hours after the start of the glucose drink. Both samples should be sent to an accredited laboratory for estimation of plasma glucose. Interpretation of the results of the OGTT test is provided in Table 1.3.

DISEASE PROCESSES OF TYPE 2 DIABETES MELLITUS

DEFECTS RESPONSIBLE FOR TYPE 2 DIABETES

The chronic hyperglycaemia of type 2 diabetes results from diverse and progressive disease processes that cause:

- defects in the ability of pancreatic beta (β) cells to secrete insulin (β-cell dysfunction)
- defects in the ability of insulin to inhibit hepatic glucose production and to promote glucose utilisation (insulin resistance).

TABLE 1.3 Interpretation of the oral glucose tolerance test (The Expert Committee 2003a, b)

Based on plasma venous glucose	Fasting (no caloric intake for 8 hours)	2 hours post 75 g glucose load
Diabetes mellitus	7.0 mmol/l or greater	11.1 mmol/l or greater
Impaired glucose tolerance	–	7.8 to 11.0 mmol/l
Impaired fasting glucose	6.1 to 6.9 mmol/l	–
Normal glucose homeostasis	6.0 mmol/l or less	7.7 mmol/l or less

In type 2 diabetes, both of these defects coexist and both can be caused by a plethora of genetic or environmental factors. Most commonly, type 2 diabetes appears to be inherited as a polygenic trait, with environmental factors also involved, often at a very young age.

Secretion of insulin, in response to rising blood glucose levels, occurs in **two** phases in healthy individuals:

1. The first (early acute) phase consists of a rapid rise in insulin immediately after an increase in blood glucose levels. This insulin is thought to originate from a small pre-formed reserve pool of insulin stored within the beta cells.
2. The second (late) phase response consists of a more gradual rise in insulin levels. The on-going biosynthesis of newly formed insulin in this phase occurs during the time that blood glucose levels are elevated.

Early in type 2 diabetes, β-cells begin to lose their initial response of increased insulin secretion ("first phase"). Sustained hyperglycaemia reduces β-cell function by "glucose toxicity". With progression of the disease, the loss of first-phase secretion leads to early post-prandial hyperglycaemia, exaggerated late ("second-phase") insulin secretion and late post-meal hypoglycaemia. Insulin secretory pulses become abnormal under basal conditions. The loss of first-phase insulin secretion, which leads to post-prandial glucose "spikes", is associated with an increased risk of cardiovascular disease.

In insulin resistance, insulin is unable to produce its usual effects at concentrations that are effective in normal individuals. Its onset precedes the development of type 2 diabetes and may arise from a variety of genetic mutations. It is thought that the reduced action of insulin is linked closely with the cardiovascular risk factors, such as obesity, that are part of the insulin resistance syndrome (Reaven 1988).

Malnutrition *in utero* and during early infancy may be associated with an increased risk of developing type 2 diabetes later in life (the "thrifty phenotype" hypothesis) by affecting both β-cell function and insulin resistance. Regular physical exercise, when undertaken consistently from childhood, can protect against type 2 diabetes by improving insulin sensitivity.

BIOCHEMISTRY OF DIABETES COMPLICATIONS

Vascular tissues are freely permeable to glucose. Poor glycaemic control renders such tissues more vulnerable to insult, which starts insidiously and may eventually lead on to the failure of major systems. Abnormalities may occur in endothelial cells, vascular smooth muscle cells, glomeruli and mesangial cells, and cardiomyocytes. The clinical consequences of diabetic microvascular disease include visual impairment, chronic renal failure and neuropathic foot ulceration.

Four main mechanisms (not mutually exclusive) have been implicated in the pathogenesis of glucose-mediated vascular damage:

1. Non-enzymatic glycation (basis for the glycated haemoglobin assay)
2. Oxidative/reductive stress
3. Aldose reductase activation
4. Activation of diacylglycerol-protein kinase C signalling.

However, clinical complications are driven by raised blood pressure, dyslipidaemia and multiple other abnormalities, particularly those that contribute to insulin resistance. Some of these precede the onset of type 2 diabetes, by which time atheromatous changes have already been established. This is why prevention or early detection is important.

The precise pathogenesis of atheromatous change in patients with diabetes may vary not just between individuals, but also between sites and different calibre of arteries in the same individual. A better understanding of these mechanisms may help to identify potential therapeutic interventions, although lifestyle modification and vigorous correction of raised blood pressure and dyslipidaemia must remain central to reducing cardiovascular risk.

INTERMEDIATE HYPERGLYCAEMIC CONDITIONS

The term "pre-diabetes" has been used to categorise people with impaired glucose metabolism, but who are not diabetic. Many, but not all, progress to diabetes. The WHO term "intermediate hyperglycaemia" may be more accurate. Whichever term is used, identification followed by appropriate interventions (particularly aimed at optimising lifestyle) can achieve real benefit for this group.

IMPAIRED GLUCOSE TOLERANCE AND IMPAIRED FASTING GLUCOSE

These terms are not interchangeable and do not define identical groups of individuals. The rationale for establishing these intermediate categories of impaired glucose regulation is based on their value in predicting cardiovascular risk (IGT) and future diabetes mellitus (IFG).

Impaired glucose tolerance (IGT) refers to a glucose metabolic state that is intermediate between normal glucose homeostasis and diabetes mellitus. IGT **only** applies to a plasma glucose level in the range of 7.8 to 11.0 mmol/l **at 2 hours after**

a 75 g glucose load. Patients can be labelled as having IGT only from an OGTT. Individuals with IGT are at increased risk of developing macrovascular disease. IGT progresses to type 2 diabetes in 37% at 5 years (Gillies 2007) and 50% at 10 years (Davies 2006). It is logical to regard IGT as a risk factor rather than as a disease entity, particularly as many individuals with IGT are asymptomatic and have normal plasma glucose levels in their daily lives. Some evidence suggests that the most cost-effective interventions to prevent or delay the onset of diabetes should target individuals with IGT, followed by high-risk groups.

Impaired fasting glucose (IFG) applies **only** to a **fasting plasma glucose level** in the range between a lower limit of 6.1 mmol/l (recommended by JBS2, WHO and the IDF) and an upper limit of 6.9 mmol/l. Some patients, particularly elderly or Indo-Asians, can have IFG, but fulfil the diagnostic criteria for diabetes because their 2 hour post 75 g load plasma glucose level is 11.1 mmol/l or greater. Thus, patients with IFG can have *either* diabetes *or* IGT *or* normal glucose homeostasis (based upon the 2 hour result). This has major implications for screening, because a fasting plasma glucose level below the diagnostic threshold for diabetes does not exclude current diabetes.

If IFG is defined as between 6.1 and 6.9 mmol/l, then it includes a much lower proportion of the population than is categorised as having IGT. One review found that of those who had IFG and/or IGT, 16% had both, 23% had IFG alone, and 60% had IGT alone, with significant age and gender differences between the glucose intolerance categories (Unwin et al 2002). IFG and IGT may be different metabolic states. Although the ADA has recommended a reduced lower limit for IFG to 5.6 mmol/l is, on balance, a better predictor for cardiovascular and metabolic outcomes (The Expert Committee 2003a), other guidance (WHO/IDF, JBS2, NICE/NSF still recommends that the lower limit should remain at 6.1 mmol/l (WHO/IDF 2006).

There has been considerable research into the factors that increase the likelihood of an individual with intermediate hyperglycaemia developing diabetes. It is also interesting to look earlier in the natural history at factors that may cause glucose intolerance. Smoking is thought to increase insulin resistance, but the evidence is inconclusive as to whether smoking is an independent risk factor for the development of diabetes. The CARDIA study found that, in young individuals with normal glucose tolerance, both active and passive smoking were associated (more so in whites) with the development of glucose intolerance (Houston et al 2006).

METABOLIC SYNDROME

Insulin resistance is associated with a collection of abnormal risk factors (obesity, impaired glucose tolerance, hypertension and dyslipidaemia) and is now recognised as a major underlying contributor to increased coronary heart disease (CHD) mortality. *Metabolic syndrome* is a defined cluster of abnormal cardiovascular risk factors; it doubles cardiovascular disease (CVD) mortality, trebles the onset of CVD events (Carr et al 2004), and predicts the development of not only type 2 diabetes, but also obstructive/sleep airways disease, gall stones, some cancers and chronic kidney disease.

The two major previous definitions of metabolic syndrome were from:

- the WHO (including evidence of insulin resistance and measurement of fasting insulin)
- the National Cholesterol Education Program (presence of three from the following clinical criteria: BP > 130/85, HDL-C < 1.04 mmol/l in men or < 1.29 mmol/l in women, TG > 1.69 mmol/l, fasting glucose > 5.6 mmol/l or abdominal obesity).

In 2005, the International Diabetes Foundation (IDF) proposed a new definition for metabolic syndrome for clinical use (set out in Table 1.4) that avoids the technical difficulties associated with insulin measurement (International Diabetes Federation 2005).

TABLE 1.4 International Diabetes Federation (IDF) definition of metabolic syndrome (IDF 2005)

Parameter	Qualifications
In all cases:	
Central obesity (waist circumference)	In men: ≥94 cm in Europids, Sub-Saharan Africans and Arabs ≥90 cm in South Asians and Chinese ≥85 cm in Japanese
	In women: ≥80 cm in all populations, except ≥90 cm in Japanese
Any 2 of the following 4:	
Raised triglyceride level	≥1.7 mmol/l OR specific treatment for this lipid abnormality
Reduced HDL-C levels	≤0.9 mmol/l in males or ≥1.1 mmol/l in females OR specific treatment for this lipid abnormality
Raised blood pressure	Systolic ≥130 mmHg or diastolic ≥80 mmHg OR treatment of previously diagnosed hypertension
Raised fasting plasma glucose	≥5.6 mmol/l (OGTT recommended to confirm diabetes) OR previously diagnosed **type 2 diabetes**

OGTT: oral glucose tolerance test

Epidemiological data about the metabolic syndrome are not entirely reliable due to the use of different definitions, but the prevalence varies amongst different ethnic groups, ranging from 22 to 39% of the adult population. It is commoner in an Indo-Asian population: a BMI greater than $23\,kg/m^2$ in Indo-Asians (as compared to $25\,kg/m^2$ in white Caucasians), is now thought to indicate increased CVD risk in this population, subject to the occasional confusion of obesity with being overweight (Hanif et al 2002).

Although the presence of metabolic syndrome does "predict" CVD events, there is no evidence that its criteria enhance the estimation of CVD risk in either diabetic or non-diabetic populations beyond existing tools, such as the New Zealand tables. However, the criteria associated with metabolic syndrome, particularly increased waist circumference, are better predictors of the development of type 2 diabetes (Sattar 2006).

Although no data are yet available from any large intervention trials in primary care for preventing or delaying diabetes or CVD in people with metabolic syndrome, there are good reasons for managing metabolic syndrome aggressively, addressing all relevant cardiovascular risk factors:

- Metabolic syndrome is clearly associated with a much greater risk of developing either CHD or type 2 diabetes or both.
- Its constituent adverse risk factors are also associated with increased cardiovascular mortality and morbidity, the result being often greater than additive.
- Metabolic syndrome itself is a significant predictor of total and cardiovascular mortality (Sundström et al 2006).
- If these constituent factors are properly addressed, then mortality and morbidity are delayed or reduced significantly.
- Many of the interventions involve improving lifestyle, where successful change is known to be beneficial for more than CVD prevention.

PREVALENCE OF TYPE 2 DIABETES

CURRENT PREVALENCE

Estimating the prevalence of type 2 diabetes mellitus risks underestimation, because many type 2 patients are asymptomatic, and these individuals and/or health-care professionals may not always recognise the symptoms of hyperglycaemia. Some of the attempts to estimate the prevalence of diabetes are listed in Table 1.5.

The National Diabetes Audit (NDA) has used the estimates for England produced by the PBS Diabetes Population Prevalence Model for 2001 and predicted for 2010, with adjustments for age, gender, ethnicity, social deprivation and district. The PBS model's overall estimate for the prevalence of diabetes in 2001 of 4.37% was higher than other estimates (YHPHO 2005). In 2005 the estimated prevalence of *all* diabetes (diagnosed

TABLE 1.5 Estimates of the prevalence of diabetes mellitus in the UK

Year	Organisation	Numbers	Prevalence (%)
1996	DARTS (Morris et al 1997)	1 060 000 with type 2 disease (extrapolated to the UK population)	1.93 (all diabetes) (89.2% of these being type 2)
1998	GPRD (Newnham et al 2002)	1 150 000 in England and Wales (all types)	Age-standardised prevalence of 2.23 per 100 males and 1.64 per 100 females
2000	NICE (NICE 2000)	800 000 with type 2 disease in England and Wales	2.4 (80% type 2) of adult population
2000	DARTS		2.51 (in Tayside)
2001	PBS model (YHPHO 2005)	2 146 627 with types 1 + 2 in England	4.37
2003	Diabetes UK (Diabetes in the UK 2004)	1 530 000	3
2004–2005	QMAS		3.544
2005	PBS model (Kingdom & Ferguson 2006)	2 350 000 with types 1 + 2 in England	4.67
2010 prediction	PBS model (YHPHO 2005)		5.05

and undiagnosed) in England was 4.67% or 2 350 000 persons (Kingdom & Ferguson 2006).

One of the quality indicators for the GMS contract is that each practice should keep a diabetic register: indicator DM1 in 2004–2006; now DM19 (see Appendix 3). Data from the monitoring process provided a "raw" national prevalence, based on the number of diabetics identified in every practice, of 3.544% in 2005, lower than the PBS model, indicating that there is still a substantial number of "missing" diabetics (about one-quarter of those with diabetes).

FUTURE PREVALENCE

It is predicted that the prevalence of type 2 diabetes will continue to increase rapidly. It has been estimated that the worldwide prevalence of type 2 diabetes will more than double from 98.9 million in 1994 to 215 million by 2010 (Amos et al 1997).

FACTORS THAT AFFECT THE PREVALENCE OF TYPE 2 DIABETES

Ethnic origin

The prevalence is particularly high in populations that have changed from a traditional to a modern life-style, such as migrant Afro-Caribbeans and Indo-Asians in the UK. Indo-Asians are not a homogeneous group, with the greatest prevalence being in Pakistanis, then in Bangladeshis and finally in Indians. For the year 2001 the PBS model estimated the prevalence of type 1 and 2 diabetes to be 6.6% in those from a South Asian background, 5.6% in those from a Black background and 4.2% in those of White origin.

Age

Most subjects are diagnosed after 40 years of age. However, a younger age of onset is now occurring more frequently, especially in certain high-prevalence ethnic groups, such as Indo-Asians and Afro-Caribbeans, and in individuals with very adverse factors for insulin resistance (i.e. obesity, sedentary lifestyle and unhealthy diet). Maturity onset diabetes of the young (MODY) syndromes, which involve genetic defects of β-cell function, are classified separately from type 2 diabetes.

For 2001, the PBS model estimated the prevalence of diabetes in England to be:

- 0.33% in those aged less than 30 years
- 3.3% in those aged 30 to 59 years
- 13.8% in those aged more than 60 years.

Gender

For 2001 the PBS model estimated the prevalence to be higher in women (1.28 million or 5.07%) than in men (869 000 or 3.6%).

Obesity

Obesity, especially truncal, is associated closely with type 2 diabetes. The risk increases as the BMI rises. Obesity is more likely to occur with the wrong diet and lack of physical exercise. Eating less and exercising more are at the core of programmes to delay or prevent the onset of type 2 diabetes. Four cases of type 2 diabetes in very obese (BMI greater than 35 kg/m^2) white adolescents were reported by Drake et al in 2002, and widely publicised in the lay press. Forty to 50% of new-onset diabetes in American children is now type 2 (Beers et al 2006). This frightening phenomenon, likely to become more common in the future, increases the priority to resource and to implement wide-ranging effective health education programmes aimed at preventing type 2 diabetes.

Deprivation

Deprivation is associated with a higher prevalence in both sexes aged 35 to 74 years (Newnham et al 2002), although it is unclear whether this is independent of the above factors. The PBS model estimated the prevalence of diabetes to be 35% higher than the mean in the most socio-economically deprived fifth of the English population.

CONSEQUENCES OF TYPE 2 DIABETES MELLITUS

DIABETIC CONTROL, MORTALITY AND COMPLICATIONS

The diagnosis of type 2 diabetes mellitus has a profoundly adverse effect on morbidity and mortality. The long-term complications are mostly commonly vascular in origin and can be divided into macrovascular (ischaemic heart disease, cerebrovascular disease, and peripheral arterial disease) or microvascular (retinopathy, nephropathy and neuropathy).

In its 2004 report, Diabetes UK listed some truly frightening statistics (Diabetes in the UK 2004):

- Reduced life expectancy by up to 10 years in type 2 diabetics.
- Evidence of complications at diagnosis in 50% of type 2 diabetics.
- In the UK diabetics spend 1.1 million days in hospital every year.
- Cardiovascular disease will be the cause of death in 80% of diabetics.
- Diabetics are two to three times more likely to have a stroke.
- 1000 diabetics start kidney dialysis every year in the UK.
- Diabetes is the leading cause of blindness in people of working age in the UK.
- The rate of lower limb amputation in diabetics is 15 times higher than in people without diabetes.

Overall, 5-year mortality in type 2 diabetics increases two- to threefold and age-adjusted life expectancy is reduced by 5 to 10 years compared to the general population (Panzram 1987), with cardiovascular disease being the predominant cause of mortality.

The adverse effects of sustained hyperglycaemia and poor management on mortality and morbidity in type 2 diabetes have been studied extensively. The UKPDS has now identified poor glycaemic control among the risk factors for coronary artery disease in type 2 diabetics (Turner et al 1998). The UKPDS also demonstrated that improving glycaemic control significantly reduced the risk of microvascular complications (e.g. retinopathy, nephropathy), with lesser reductions in macrovascular disease (e.g. CHD, major stroke) and no effect on diabetes-related mortality in type 2 diabetics (UKPDS 1998a, Stratton et al 2000).

As many type 2 patients at diagnosis have complications, particularly vascular, and/or adverse cardiovascular risk factors, early diagnosis (including targeted screening) and high-quality management can improve their future well-being.

FINANCIAL CONSEQUENCES OF TYPE 2 DIABETES

Several attempts have been made to ascertain precisely how much is spent both directly and indirectly on diabetes care.

In 2002, the Diabetes NSF estimated that the NHS spent £3.5 billion per year on treating diabetes and its complications (Department of Health 2002). Since then the actual costs will have increased, due to economic and health-care inflation and to the rising prevalence of type 2 diabetes. T2ARDIS estimated that diabetes was responsible for 5% of the total NHS expenditure (British Diabetic Association 2000). The prevalence of type 2 diabetes, with its associated morbidity and mortality, continues to increase, as do its costs and the pressures on those responsible for financing health care. Diabetes UK predicted that the proportion of NHS expenditure on diabetes will rise to 10% by 2011 (Diabetes in the UK 2004).

The UKPDS calculated the annual manpower cost of implementing its findings for glycaemic and blood pressure control in patients with type 2 diabetes to be £264 per patient in 1998 (UKPDS 1998a, b).

The **T**ype **2** Diabetes: **A**ccounting for a major **R**esource **D**emand in **S**ociety in the UK (T2ARDIS) project looked at the financial impact of type 2 diabetes and presented its results to Diabetes UK's Annual Professional Conference in March 2000 (British Diabetic Association 2000). T2ARDIS calculated that the average annual cost of treating each person with type 2 diabetes incurred direct costs to the country of £2152, comprising:

- £1738 (81%) to the NHS, the total annual cost being £2 billion, 4.7% of the total NHS expenditure, with hospitalisation consuming more than 40% of diabetes-related NHS expenditure.
- £285 (13%) borne by the private individual.
- £129 (6%) to the social services. Over 75% of social services costs for people with type 2 diabetes are associated with residential and nursing care.

T2ARDIS also showed that the presence of both microvascular and macrovascular complications in an individual increased the average NHS costs in the calculation above fivefold, personal expenditure threefold, and social services costs fourfold.

Published in 2002, the CODE-2 study gathered data on 7000 type 2 diabetics from eight European studies: it estimated the average annual cost per patient to be £1934, of which 55% could be attributed to hospital admissions and 7% to the cost of blood glucose-lowering medication (Jonsson 2002); these estimates are not too dissimilar to T2ARDIS.

At Diabetes UK's Annual Professional Conference in April 2005, Professor Rhys Williams presented predictions that, by 2025, diabetes care worldwide could cost between US$153 and 286 billions, accounting for 7.5 to 13.5% of total health-care costs: a terrifying prospect.

Wanless estimated that the additional annual cost of implementing fully the Diabetes NSF in England by 2010–2011 would be £600 million; however, an annual saving of £200 million would result from measures that reduce the medical effects of diabetes (by prevention, earlier detection or improved care to reduce complications).

SCREENING FOR TYPE 2 DIABETES MELLITUS

GENERAL POINTS AND DEFINITIONS

Diagnostic testing and screening are two distinct processes. In diabetes, although both use the same clinical tests (blood glucose measurements), diagnostic tests are performed when an individual exhibits suggestive clinical features of diabetes, whereas screening aims to identify asymptomatic people who may already have or be at imminent risk of developing diabetes. The initial screening process may be followed by the appropriate diagnostic tests.

Screening for diabetes in primary care is an important public health issue. Despite the findings of important studies, such as the recent DHDS, there are still large gaps in the evidence needed to inform the decisions that must be made about any screening programme.

HOW STRONG IS THE CASE FOR SCREENING FOR TYPE 2 DIABETES?

Since setting up and implementing any screening programme can be a major undertaking with considerable costs, it is necessary to be able to evaluate the benefits of any proposal against recognised criteria (Davies 1997, The Expert Committee 2003a). The role of the National Screening Committee (NSC) is to provide advice about established and newly proposed screening programmes, with the aim of evaluating these against specified criteria, published in 1998 and divided into four areas: the condition, the test, the treatment and the screening programme (National Screening Committee 1998).

While the NSC crirteria are primarily designed to evaluate the cost-effectiveness of a screening programme, it may be more useful at practice level to evaluate the benefits of screening against established and recognised criteria (The Expert Committee 2003a). These can be summarised as follows:

1. *The prevalence of the disease in the population to be screened must be sufficiently large to make mass screening practical.*
   The UK prevalence of diabetes in 2005 was estimated to be at least 4.67% and is rising. This prevalence is greater with increasing age, particular ethnicity and/or the presence of one or more other risk factors (hypertension, obesity, family history of diabetes) (Lawrence et al 2001).
2. *The disease must be clearly defined to allow an accurate diagnosis.*
   There are diagnostic criteria for type 2 diabetes.
3. *There should be evidence that the disease is undiagnosed in a significant proportion of individuals, so that a prompt early diagnosis is not inevitable in most of these cases.*
   It is estimated that about a quarter of diabetics are undiagnosed. There is good evidence that most type 2 diabetics have had their disease at least 4 to 7 years prior to clinical diagnosis (Harris et al 1992). Complications are already evident in many patients at diagnosis.
4. *Early diagnosis of the disease must result in improved outcomes, including disease treatment and reduced impact of complications.*
   At least one-third of patients with type 2 diabetes have at least one complication present at diagnosis (UKDIABS 2000). However, type 2 diabetics identified by screening have:

- a significant cluster of cardiovascular risk factors, which can be improved by early intervention (Davies et al 1996)
- a lower prevalence of microvascular complications at diagnosis (UKDIABS 2000)
- a lower risk of death than in known type 2 diabetes patients after 4 years in a UK study (Croxson et al 1994).

Patients found to have IGT may benefit from interventions to reduce both their risk of becoming diabetic in the future and of their existing propensity to develop cardiovascular disease. Ultimately, the practice must be able to offer high-quality, appropriate and effective care on a consistent basis to newly diagnosed diabetics.

Diagnosis should not cause physical harm. There are numerous interventions in diabetes for which the benefits outweigh harm, although any intervention carries some degree of risk.

5. *The screening test(s) used must be readily available and must have an acceptable specificity, sensitivity and predictive value in the population to be screened.*

Reliable blood-glucose estimation is readily available by sending samples to an accredited local chemical pathology laboratory. The three methods of diagnosing diabetes (random, fasting and OGTT) have a high sensitivity (i.e. the likelihood of a positive result in patients with disease) and positive predictive value, because they define the disease, which is a lifelong diagnosis. However, a negative OGTT has a higher specificity (i.e. the likelihood of a negative result in patients without disease) than a negative fasting or random plasma glucose, because a proportion of diabetics can be missed by the latter two screening tests. The predictive value of a negative result is not conclusive, since currently non-diabetic individuals, particularly those from higher risk groups, may develop diabetes in the future. A result that demonstrates IGT, although negative for diabetes, does predict an increased future risk of developing diabetes.

6. *The screening test(s) used must be acceptable to individuals being screened, and not cause significant adverse effects.*

Venepuncture is invasive, but low risk when performed competently. Most would probably find it acceptable, provided informed consent is obtained. Screening, however, may cause anxiety, which needs to be minimised.

7. *Case finding and treatment must be cost-effective, in relation to health expenditure as a whole.*

This is unlikely if screening the general population solely for diabetes (Goodyer 2006). In addition to a lower yield of new cases, whole-population screening requires considerable resources. One study calculated the workload as 1 hour per week for a year to screen 620 patients during that period (Lawrence et al 2001). However, a screening programme that recruited well elderly Americans found that the presence of certain factors (age, gender, ethnicity, raised BMI, greater waist: hip ratio, hypertension) increased the yield to as much as one new case of diabetes diagnosed for every six individuals screened (Franse et al 2001).

Targeted screening of "high-risk" groups would require less resource and produce a higher yield (thus, be more practical) than screening the whole population. If additional information needed to estimate cardiovascular risk was gathered at screening, then all screened individuals, even the majority who screen negative for diabetes, could benefit from this estimation, particularly if interventions are available to reduce this risk.

8. *Facilities and resources must be available to treat newly diagnosed cases.*

Screening is likely to be undertaken using existing staff and facilities. It is unlikely that additional resources will be provided in the near future, either for screening or for the treatment of new cases; these will need to be found from existing resources.

9. *Screening should be a systematic on-going process.*

It should not merely be an isolated one-time effort. Depending upon what the National Screening Committee recommends, any screening programme will need to be managed, with an agreed set of quality assurance standards. Primary care is well placed to develop the accurate population and disease registers required to identify at-risk subjects, and to undertake regularly both recall and screening tests, provided that adequate systems are in place and maintained.

In 2001 it was argued that the case for whole-population screening for diabetes could not be made (Wareham & Griffin 2001). In the light of current evidence, the case for a cost-effective screening programme can be made only if either:

- a selected "high-risk" population is targeted

    or

- other parameters contributing to cardiovascular risk are included in the screening.

PRACTICAL ISSUES IN SCREENING FOR TYPE 2 DIABETES

Any practice seeking to screen a population for type 2 diabetes needs to consider its answers to five practical questions:

1. Who to screen?
2. Which screening method(s) should be used?
3. How often to screen?
4. Should anything else be done at the time of screening?
5. Is the practice able to provide high-quality care to newly diagnosed diabetics without detriment to other patients?

Additional evidence is required to resolve fully the uncertainties that surround the first three questions, a point recognised by the Diabetes NSF.

Who to screen?

Instead of whole-population screening, the current consensus is for a targeted screening approach that concentrates on those at "high risk" with:

- previous IGT, metabolic syndrome (particularly obese or those with large waist circumference) or gestational diabetes (or high-birth-weight babies)

- existing cardiovascular disease
- strong family history of diabetes, i.e. first-degree relative
- increased-risk ethnicity, particularly older Indo-Asians and Afro-Caribbeans
- recurrent or major sepsis, or peripheral skin breakdown
- autoimmune endocrinopathies (e.g. primary hypothyroidism) or organ-specific disorders (e.g. polycystic ovary disease).

It is sensible to create a register of these "high-risk" individuals to facilitate recall.

Which screening method to use?

The logistics and greater resource demands of the OGTT render it unsuitable to be undertaken as the first-line test on a large scale in primary care. Therefore, a preliminary screening test needs to be performed to identify those who require an OGTT, as a second stage. The two tests that might serve as a first-stage screen are:

1. Fasting plasma glucose
2. Glycosylated haemoglobin (HbA1c).

Fasting plasma glucose test is less sensitive and specific, but may be a sensible compromise as the initial screening test. However, fasting plasma glucose has a reduced specificity because many individuals, particularly Indo-Asians, with a non-diabetic fasting level will have a diabetic level at 2 hours post glucose load. The STAR study suggests that a reasonable cut off for Indo-Asians under the age of 40 years is below 5.9 mmol/l. For Indo-Asians aged 40 to 75 years, an HbA1c below 6.2% is a reasonable cut-off for excluding diabetes (Davies 2006). Urine testing is simple, quick and cheap, but does not fulfil the diagnostic criteria for diabetes and a raised renal threshold may miss a diabetic blood glucose level.

In the event of diagnostic uncertainty or if the individual being screened is considered to be at high risk of diabetes, then an OGTT should be performed.

How often to screen?

Diabetes UK recommends (but supporting evidence is not cast-iron) that screening should not be performed more often than every 5 years in subjects with no risk factors, and no more often than every 3 years in those with one risk factor.

Should anything else be done at the time of screening?

For greater cost-effectiveness, individuals who are invited for screening should have a cardiovascular risk assessment that includes also blood pressure, lipids, smoking status and waist circumference.

Is the practice able to provide high-quality care to newly diagnosed diabetics without detriment to other patients?

While recognising the strong arguments in favour of targeted screening for diabetes, a practice should not forget that:

- screening will require additional resources, particularly of staff time
- the newly diagnosed diabetic patient should receive high-quality, appropriate and effective care on a consistent basis
- the delivery of care to other patients with existing diabetes and/or other significant problems must be maintained and not suffer when additional tasks are taken on.

THE LIKELY FUTURE SHAPE OF DIABETES SCREENING PROGRAMMES

The Diabetes Heart Disease and Stroke (DHDS) Project was set up to explore these practical issues. In its 2006 report, the overall "pick-up" rate for newly diagnosed diabetics was 4.3% of those screened (Goodyer 2006), but the rate varied, being higher in those populations where the prevelance of diabetes is greater. Although the project did not evaluate cost-effectiveness, the results do not support this in a screening programme searching solely for new cases of diabetes in a general population; rather, the screening for diabetes in a general population is best incorporated into a general vascular risk assessment.

This point both informs and underlies the Department of Health's 2006 White Paper (DoH 2006) which proposes health MOTs at various stages of life. At the time of writing, a diabetes screening programme is unlikely to stand alone, but would be incorporated into a population-wide assessment, probably at significant age milestones (i.e. 40, 50 and 60 years), of parameters (that may include waist circumference, blood pressure, fasting lipids and glucose) which will identify a subset with metabolic syndrome that may need more frequent (every 3 years?) fasting blood glucose checks.

Ultimately, any systematic and sustained programme requires sufficient additional resources for screening, diagnostic tests and treatment; and their provision must be balanced against other demands made upon the practice. A practice's decisions need to be based upon what is most feasible, both logistically and clinically.

PREVENTION OF TYPE 2 DIABETES MELLITUS

WHY PREVENT TYPE 2 DIABETES?

NSF ◀
1
3

The predicted rise in prevalence makes all the greater the need to consider and to implement effective preventive strategies. Not all people are at equal risk of developing diabetes. Certain factors, such as age, ethnic origin and family history, are unalterable. However, many individuals who develop type 2 diabetes have a less than optimal lifestyle, over which they do have control. Factors associated with both increased cardiovascular risk and greater insulin resistance are already present in British children, particularly of Indo-Asian origin (Whincup et al 2002). A healthier diet and increased exercise reduces insulin resistance and cardiovascular risk.

POSSIBLE INTERVENTIONS TO PREVENT TYPE 2 DIABETES: EVIDENCE BASE

A number of published studies demonstrate that type 2 diabetes in high-risk individuals can be prevented either by improving lifestyle or by prescribing medication.

Modifying lifestyle

The Da Qing IGT and Diabetes Study (China), which followed up individuals with IGT over 6 years, showed a reduction by at least one-third of the incidence of new diabetes with either diet or exercise interventions or both (Pan et al 1997).

The Finnish Diabetes Prevention Study Group, followed up overweight individuals with IGT over a mean of 3.2 years, and compared "individualised" counselling aimed at reducing weight, modifying diet and increasing physical activity against controls. The cumulative incidence of new diabetes was reduced by 58% in the intervention group, or one case of diabetes was prevented for every 22 overweight individuals with impaired glucose tolerance "treated" for 1 year (Tuomilehto et al 2001). The benefits were sustained (APR 3.1%; RRR 43%) during a median follow-up of 3 years after the intervention was discontinued (Lindstrom 2006).

The Diabetes Prevention Program (DPP) in the USA, followed up "high-risk" subjects over a mean of 2.8 years, and compared three arms: standard lifestyle recommendations plus placebo, standard lifestyle recommendations plus metformin, and an intensive programme of lifestyle modification (16 lessons covering diet, exercise and behaviour modification). The reduction in incidence of new cases of diabetes was 31% in the metformin group (treat 41.7 subjects for 1 year to prevent one new case) and 58% in the intensive programme group (treat 20.7 subjects for 1 year to prevent one new case) (Diabetes Prevention Program Research Group 2002).

To apply any of the above programmes on a sustained basis to a large population will require considerable effort and resources. However, the evidence does support modifications of lifestyle:

- increased levels of physical activity, along the lines of 30 minutes of "moderate" exercise (e.g. brisk walking) at least five times per week
- reduced fat and limited calorific intake

with the aim of achieving and maintaining weight reduction, which has considerable health benefits beyond preventing type 2 diabetes.

Medication

Any drug shown to be effective in preventing diabetes could potentially create a huge market for pharmaceutical companies. Even if proved effective, the colossal financial costs of treating large populations with some of these drugs may be prohibitive.

The following studies investigated drug therapy to prevent diabetes using different classes of glucose-lowering agents:

- The DPP (cited above) demonstrated a reduction in incidence of type 2 diabetes in high-risk subjects who used *metformin*, but lifestyle changes were even more effective as prevention (Diabetes Prevention Program Research Group 2002).
- In a multicentre randomised trial, Study to Prevent NIDDM (STOP-NIDDM), conversion of impaired glucose tolerance into type 2 diabetes was less in patients treated with *acarbose* than with placebo. However, 31% of the patients allocated to the acarbose group discontinued treatment early (Chiasson et al 2002). The use of acarbose is limited by frequent gastrointestinal side effects.
- In the Troglitazone in Prevention of Diabetes (TRIPOD) study, Hispanic women with "recent" gestational diabetes were randomised to receive either placebo or *troglitazone* (a glitazone now withdrawn from commercial sale). In the treated group there was a 56% relative reduction in the incidence of diabetes (Buchanan et al 2005).

In addition:

- *Orlistat* was added to lifestyle change in a group with BMI equal to or greater than 30 kg/m^2, with or without IGT, in the XENical in the prevention of Diabetes in Obese Subjects (XENDOS) study. After 4 years of treatment, the addition of orlistat corresponded to a 45% risk reduction of new diabetes in the IGT group, with no effect observed in those without IGT (Torgerson et al 2004).

Finally, there are data to suggest that blockade of the renin-angiotensin system may prevent diabetes:

- An incidental finding in the Heart Outcomes Prevention Evaluation (HOPE) trial was the lower rate of new diagnosis of diabetes in vascular high-risk patients aged over 55 years treated with the ACE inhibitor *ramipril* (Yusuf et al 2001). In the Diabetes Reduction Assessment with Ramipril and Rosiglitazone Medication (DREAM) study, rosiglitazone, unlike ramipril when compared to placebo, reduced significantly (hazard ratio 0.40, 95% Cl 0.35–0.46) the risk of patients with impaired fasting glucose or IGT developing diabetes. Although the study was well conducted, the results need to be interpreted and applied with caution, as rosiglitazone did increase fluid retention and heart failure and it is still an expensive drug being used to treat here something for which changes in lifestyles are still the mainstay.
- In the Losartan Intervention for Endpoint Reduction in Hypertension (LIFE) study, which looked at cardiovascular morbidity and mortality in patients with essential hypertension and left ventricular hypertrophy and compared treatment using the ARB *losartan* with *atenolol*, new-onset diabetes was less common in the losartan-treated group (Dählof et al 2002).
- In the VALUE study, although designed to evaluate cardiovascular outcomes in high-risk hypertensive subjects, new-onset diabetics was significantly less in the ARB *valsartan* treatment group compared with the CCB *amlodipine* treatment group (Julius et al 2004).
- A recent meta-analysis of 12 RCTs found that, in high-risk individuals (pre-diabetic conditions, such as IFG, metabolic syndrome), ACE inhibitors and ARBs were associated with relative risk reductions in the incidence of newly diagnosed diabetes by 25% in the pooled analysis (Abuissa et al 2005). However, further research is needed to determine the mechanism of action.

The HOPE and LIFE studies found that inhibition of the renin-angiotensin system may improve glucose tolerance. The LIFE study authors suggested an effect on insulin resistance, but other hypotheses suggest an increased insulin secretory response, either by inducing a raised pancreatic islet blood flow to secure a better early insulin response (Carlsson et al 1998) or as a result of the higher serum potassium levels associated with ACE-inhibitor use augmenting insulin secretion (Santoro et al 1992).

However, a recent systematic review concluded that, despite data that some drugs lowered the incidence of diabetes compared to placebo, no single pharmacological intervention can be definitively recommended for diabetes prevention. Further research is needed, using studies designed with the incidence of diabetes as the primary outcome and of sufficient duration to differentiate between real prevention and the delay or masking of the condition (Padwal et al 2005). Whilst the benefits of lifestyle changes may last beyond the period of intervention, it is unclear whether the benefit of medication is sustained. Although evidence supports the effectiveness of both lifestyle and pharmacological interventions in reducing the risk of IGT progressing to type 2 diabetes (Gillies 2007), selecting the optimal intervention requires careful consideration of benefit vs. harm, patient preference, likely concordance, available resources and other issues that are, as yet, unresolved.

DEVELOPING POLICIES THAT TACKLE PREVENTION: ISSUES THAT NEED TO BE CONSIDERED

Societies and their health services will need to look at implementing a range of measures targeted at individuals to whole populations. Successful health education requires collaboration between disparate agencies with a unity of purpose, from appropriate government policies down to practice level. Health professionals have an important role, but are not the only players here. Government policy is reflected in Chapter 6 of the NSF Diabetes' Strategy, which refers to national initiatives and best-practice models that tackle diet, physical activity and smoking cessation, particularly in schools and/or deprived areas (DoH 2002).

The huge demand placed upon finite resources (financial and human) is one of the main barriers to applying and sustaining successfully any of the above interventions to a large population. The practical compromise may be to give priority to proven interventions in those individuals most likely to benefit.

Attempts to change an individual's behaviour raise the potential dilemmas that surround patient empowerment. The concept is laudable and may often enhance effective disease management; however, individuals have the right to make choices that ultimately may cause them harm. Lifestyles are largely the result of choices made by individuals. Any intervention to alter these must respect each individual's right to make decisions and must assess each individual's willingness to change.

Another challenge for health professionals and organisations is to develop clear and equitable policies in response to patient demands for available interventions that may lack full clinical justification or affordability within a limited budget.

▶ KEY POINTS

- Type 2 diabetes is characterised by a chronic elevation of blood glucose, which results from defects in insulin secretion, insulin action (also known as insulin resistance) or both.

- The criterion for diagnosis is a plasma glucose level either randomly of 11.1 mmol/l or greater *or* fasting of 7.0 mmol/l or greater *or* 2 hours post 75 g glucose load of 11.1 mmol/l or greater from an OGTT – on a single occasion if symptomatic or on two separate occasions if asymptomatic.

- Impaired glucose tolerance is a significant predictor of diabetes and macrovascular disease.

- It is estimated that 4.67% of the adult population had diabetes mellitus in 2005 and approximately 90% of these have type 2 disease, with the prevalence set to rise.

- Ethnicity (especially Indo-Asian), age and obesity are associated with increased prevalence.

- Age-adjusted life expectancy in type 2 diabetics is reduced by 5 to 10 years compared to the general population, with 58% of all mortality in type 2 patients caused by cardiovascular disease alone. Poor glycaemic control increases risk.

- Approximately 5% of the total health-care expenditure in the NHS is for the care of diabetics, predicted to rise to 10% by 2011. Diabetes complications are a major cause of these high costs.

- Factors associated with increased cardiovascular risk and greater insulin resistance are already present in British children, particularly those of Indo-Asian origin. Individuals can reduce their insulin resistance by eating a healthier diet and by undertaking increased appropriate exercise.

- Whole-population screening for diabetes is not cost-effective: targeted screening for diabetes with cardiovascular risk assessment is. Early detection of the disease reduces its impact.

- Prevention or delay of diabetes can be achieved through adopting a healthier lifestyle, with some effectiveness achieved using drugs.

LIFESTYLE

OVERVIEW

Diabetes mellitus is the epitome of a chronic disease in which the goals and management extend beyond purely medical interventions "owned" by a clinician. Although "patient empowerment" has acquired more than a whiff of political correctness, it is, nevertheless, at the centre of diabetic management: the patient "owns" his disease and his lifestyle can have a major effect on morbidity and mortality.

Since lifestyle is a collection of behaviours, interventions by health-care professionals will be based upon providing suitable and effective health education. The patient's concordance with well-meant guidance depends upon persuasion that any change in his behaviour will be in his self-interest.

The components of lifestyle discussed in this section can affect morbidity and mortality not just in diabetics but in the general population. Many of the concepts and interventions discussed below may be appropriate in a non-diabetic population.

DIET OR MEDICAL NUTRITIONAL THERAPY

Medical nutritional therapy (MNT) is an essential component of diabetes management, not only in optimising glycaemic control, but also in reducing cardiovascular risk.

Diabetics no longer require a separate diet with special food products: a "healthy" diabetic diet suits most of the general population, particularly when the modification of cardiovascular risk is a priority. MNT involves balancing complex issues and needs, tailored to the lifestyle, cultural and religious customs, and to the patient's overall diabetes management.

NSF
1
7

GOALS OF MEDICAL NUTRITIONAL THERAPY IN TYPE 2 DIABETES MELLITUS

An optimal diet for a diabetic should ensure that the individual is both able and encouraged to make appropriate choices:

1. *Essential nutrition must be provided*, taking into account the special needs of the patient. Type 2 diabetics need the same essential nutrients as everyone else.
2. *The risk of developing vascular complications should be minimised* by enabling and encouraging the individual to make eating choices that help correct adverse risk factors: dyslipidaemia, hypertension, obesity, and physical inactivity.
3. *The diet should allow adaptation to metabolic problems.* Food intake in type 2 diabetics must be balanced with exercise and hypoglycaemic treatment, avoiding the twin perils of hypoglycaemia and hyperglycaemia. Most type 2 patients are overweight, and thus need to reduce their energy intake.
4. If weight loss is sought, then the *reduction of energy intake* should aim to produce a daily deficit of 500 to 1000 kcal, but not to drop below the bands of 1200–1600 kcal/day for men and of 1000–1200 kcal/day for women (ADA 2007).

ASSESSMENT OF DIET

Information gathering about diet should not be restricted to current behaviour, but should also enquire about willingness and barriers to change. An assessment may involve questioning both the patient and other members of the household, and from reviewing a food diary which the patient may be asked to keep.

A nutritional assessment might include information about the following:

- *Meal patterns:* the usual pattern of meals and snacks throughout the day. It is also important to elicit the extent to which this varies from day to day, between weekdays and weekends, and the influence of factors such as working patterns, travel and school (where applicable).
- *Food choices:* the types of and typical quantities consumed of foods that make up these meals and snacks.
- *Overall dietary balance:* how closely does the current diet correspond to "Balance of Good Health" guidelines (see below), particularly how much fruit and vegetables are consumed?
- *Nutritional adequacy:* is there a dietary surplus or deficiency?
- *Alcohol consumption:* does this exceed the safe limits?
- *Beliefs or misconceptions relating to diabetes and diet:* these might include sugar is forbidden or diabetic food products are essential.

At the end of a dietetic assessment, sufficient information should be available to help the patient set achievable dietary goals and know the optimal choices to achieve them.

BASIC DIETARY RECOMMENDATIONS

In 2003 Diabetes UK issued a comprehensive list of consensus-based recommendations for diabetics that drew upon many sources to provide detailed practical advice for professionals to implement (Connor et al 2003). These are summarised in Table 2.1. The American Diabetes Association has also published its recommendations in its annually updated guidance.

Central to MNT must be changes in the patient's behaviour. Crucial to helping to bring about change is an understanding of various aspects of health education, discussed in detail later in this section.

MODELS OF DIETARY ADVICE

Appropriate dietary advice should follow practical models that reflect current dietetic thinking. The two following models may provide a useful basis for dietary advice:

1. "The Balance of Good Health" is a nationally agreed model for dietary advice for patients with diabetes (Leicestershire Health). The model divides foods into five groups:
   - Fruit and vegetables – five portions (400 g) daily
   - Bread, other cereals and potatoes – five portions daily, prefer high-fibre kinds

TABLE 2.1 Summary of recommendations for a diabetes diet–based upon Diabetes UK 2003 (Connor et al 2003) and ADA position statement (ADA 2007)

Component	Comments
Protein	Not > 1 g per kg body weight (different for nephropathy and children)
Total fat	< 35% of energy intake
Saturated + transunsaturated fat	< 7% of energy intake with *trans* fat intake minimised
n-6 polyunsaturated fat	< 10% of energy intake
n-3 polyunsaturated fat	Eat fish, especially oily fish, 1–2 times weekly
	Fish oil supplements not recommended
cis-monounsaturated fat*	10–20%
Total carbohydrate*	45–60%
Sucrose	Up to 10% of daily energy, eaten within the context of a healthy diet
	Consider using non-nutritive sweeteners where appropriate if overweight and/or hypertriglyceridaemic
Fibre	No quantitative recommendation
	Soluble fibre has beneficial effects on glycaemic and lipid metabolism
	"Insoluble" fibre has no direct effects on glycaemic and lipid metabolism, but its high satiety content may help weight loss and is advantageous to gastrointestinal health
Vitamins and anti-oxidants	Encourage foods naturally rich in vitamins and antioxidants
	Supplements are usually not recommended (except in special circumstances) and some may be harmful
Salt	< 6 g sodium chloride per day

*combined should total 60–70% of energy intake

- Milk and dairy foods – choose lower fat alternatives
- Meat, fish and alternatives – aim for smaller portions (a maximum of two portions daily) and lower fat alternatives
- Fatty and sugary foods – reduce quantities.

2. "The Healthy Eating Pyramid" is a visual way to help translate dietary advice into practical eating habits (Krentz & Bailey 2001). Foods are divided into three strata based upon what proportion of a healthy diabetic diet they should constitute:

- Consume sparingly: minimum amounts of fats, alcohol and sugars (e.g. cakes, fried food, savoury snacks, processed meat, honey, diabetes "specialist" foods)
- Consume in moderation: small servings of protein foods (e.g. lean meat, fish, eggs, low-fat dairy products)
- Consume as the basis of diet: mainly foods rich in starch (e.g. vegetables, beans, fresh fruit, wholemeal bread, pasta, rice).

Diabetes dietetic advice should emphasise the need to space regular meals and snacks appropriately throughout the day. This will spread nutrient intake and avoid hypoglycaemia. If the daily energy intake is appropriate, the frequency of meals is not critical; however, dieticians advise eating at regular intervals and not undergoing prolonged spells without food: avoiding a "feast or famine" eating pattern. By making the mealtime an occasion to enjoy and savour food, patients may avoid abstractly consuming (possibly excess quantities of) food while focused upon another activity. Patients should be warned to avoid special diabetic products, which are often expensive and with a high fat content.

Due to recent concerns about the accuracy of food labelling in the UK, shoppers do need to pay close attention to the information provided on labels and to not accept blindly adjectives such as "healthy", "low", "high" or "restricted".

WEIGHT MANAGEMENT

(See also discussion of obesity in Chapter 4.)

To achieve a slow and progressive weight loss (1 to 2 kg per month), structured dietary advice (based upon the assessment) should be guiding and supporting the patient to make eating choices that produce a sustained energy deficit of 500 to 1000 kcal per day. These need to be tailored to the patient's own needs and preferences and combined with increased levels of physical activity.

Most people eat a fairly consistent volume of food from day to day, irrespective of its energy content. Reducing significantly total quantities may be difficult. It is better to focus upon reducing the energy content of this bulk (dietary energy density, expressed as kcal per 100 g or 100 ml of food), allowing a sufficient amount of food to be consumed for satiety, but with a lower energy yield.

Probably the most important change is to replace fat-rich foods and other dietary fat sources with starchy carbohydrate foods, maintaining nutrition. Alcohol contains 7 kcal/g, and should be restricted in a weight management programme.

DIETARY CARBOHYDRATE

The glycaemic response to foods can be affected by several factors:

- The quantity of carbohydrate consumed. This has a much greater effect upon glycaemia than the source or type of carbohydrate.
- The type of carbohydrate consumed.

- The effects of cooking or processing on food structure.
- Other meal components (fats and proteins).

Dietary carbohydrate is a source not only of energy, but also of water-soluble vitamins and minerals.

Quantity of carbohydrate

The carbohydrate intake should comprise 45–60% of total calories, but the proportion may vary according to individual factors, such as age, activity levels and weight. The total carbohydrate consumed should not normally be less than 130 g per day, since the brain and central nervous system have a minimum requirement for glucose as an energy source.

Glycaemic control can be optimised by controlling the quantity, timing and distribution of carbohydrate consumed. Educating diabetics about this can involve different approaches:

1. The "*plate method*" is suitable for patients with type 2 diabetes either not on insulin or on insulin in fixed doses. The dinner plate serves as a pie chart to demonstrate the proportions of the plate that can be covered by the different main food groups: one fifth of the total area (the smallest sector) is for meat, fish, eggs or cheese; two fifths are for the staple food (rice, pasta, bread, potatoes, etc.), and two fifths are for fruit and vegetables.
2. "*Carbohydrate counting or exchanges*" may be more suitable for those on more complex insulin regimens, such as the basal bolus, allowing patients to maintain reasonably stable plasma glucose levels during varying carbohydrate intake at mealtimes. It requires creating a meal plan (usually with dietetic advice), reading food labels and doing some calculations. Flexible insulin adjustments to a basal bolus regimen are made to match the carbohydrate in a free diet on a meal by meal basis. Carbohydrate counting may use portions equivalent of 10 to 12 g carbohydrate and the soluble insulin dose is adjusted by 1 to 3 units per portion (as in the DAFNE programme – see later in this section). There are numerous references for counting: a useful one is from the Leeds Hospitals NHS Trust, online at:
   http://www.leedsth.nhs.uk/sites/diabetes/food/CarbohydrateCountingRef.php

Reducing the total quantity of carbohydrate consumed is the basis of producing an energy deficit of between 500 and 1000 kcal/day. Very low calorie diets (VLCD) are defined as containing less than 800 kcal/day and are designed to produce more rapid weight loss in very obese individuals (BMI greater than 35 kg/m^2). However, there is no evidence that they produce better long-term results and should **only** be used under careful specialist supervision with close attention paid to glycaemic control and nutritional maintenance.

Type of carbohydrate

The terms *sugars, starch* and *fibre* are preferred to the terms simple sugars, complex and fast-acting carbohydrates, as the latter are not well defined. The glycaemic index (GI) has been devised to quantify the glycaemic effect of different foods. However, different methods of food processing and preparation, and ripeness in some cases, can alter the GI. Consuming food with a low GI has not been shown to improve glycaemic control in type 2 diabetics, but may improve the lipid profile. However, using the GI may provide additional benefit for glycaemic control beyond that observed for carbohydrate monitoring alone (ADA 2007).

Fibre-containing foods, such as whole grains, fruit and vegetables, provide vitamins, minerals and other important substances, and should be included in the diet. However, very large amounts of fibre would need to be consumed to produce metabolic improvements on glycaemia and lipid profiles. Sucrose or sucrose-containing foods should not be restricted for diabetics, but can be used in substitution for other carbohydrate sources.

DIETARY PROTEIN

Protein is an essential nutrient that provides amino acids for new tissue formation. Protein intake should constitute 15 to 20% of the total energy intake (optimally 0.8 g/kg body weight/day). Moderate hyperglycaemia can cause increased protein turnover, but, since most adults eat at least 50% more protein than required, intake should not be increased to compensate.

DIETARY FAT

Both Diabetes UK (Connor et al 2003) and the National Cholesterol Education Program (Expert Panel 2001) recommend that the total fat should not exceed 35% of the total energy intake. The most important dietary modification is to reduce the intake of saturated fat, the principal dietary determinant of serum LDL-cholesterol levels; saturated and trans-unsaturated fat should provide less than 7% (ADA 2007) or 10% (Connor et al 2003) of energy. Unfortunately, in most European countries, current intake of saturated fat is above the recommended maximum 10% of total energy intake.

The main advice should be:

1. To reduce overall quantities of fat-rich foods (e.g. cheese, butter, cream, some meats, poultry). Choose "low-fat" alternatives where possible.
2. To reduce consumption of saturated fats and substitute monounsaturated fats (e.g. olive oil and pure vegetable oil), if needed, for cooking.

Sterols and stanols of plant origin have been shown to reduce serum LDL-C levels, and are now incorporated into spreads and other fat-derived products, such as yoghurts, semi-skimmed milk, cereal bars and soft cheeses. These are marketed as adjuncts to other methods of lowering LDL-cholesterol. However, the spreads are markedly more expensive than conventional margarines, their effect on long-term cardiovascular morbidity and mortality is unknown, and their benefits may be offset by reductions in fat-soluble vitamin absorption and in plasma concentrations of the antioxidants β- and α-carotene and vitamin E. Furthermore, they may not reduce total energy intake or weight.

FIBRE

As with the general population, diabetics should benefit from consuming a range of foods containing fibre, such as fibre-rich cereals (more than 5 g of fibre/serving), fruits, vegetables and whole-grain products. These are sources of vitamins and minerals.

MICRONUTRIENTS AND ANTIOXIDANTS

Diabetics should be aware of both the importance of consuming adequate quantities of vitamins and minerals from natural sources and the potential toxicity of very large doses of these in supplements. Supplementation is indicated only in selected patient groups (e.g. elderly, those on restricted calorie diets and those with proved deficiency). Although diabetics may be in a "state of increased oxidative stress", there is no placebo-controlled trial evidence of benefit of antioxidant vitamin supplementation.

REDUCED CALORIE SWEETENERS

Reduced calorie sweeteners available include sugar alcohols (erythritol, hydrogenated starch hydrolysates, isomalt, lactitol, maltitol, mannitol, sorbitol and xylitol) and tagatose. If undertaking calorie counting, then one can subtract one-half of sugar alcohol grams from total carbohydrate grams. There is no evidence that consuming sugar alcohol will reduce energy intake significantly or improve glycaemic control over the long term.

CHROMIUM

There is still "insufficient evidence to support any of the proposed health claims for chromium supplementation" (ADA 2007).

ALCOHOLIC DRINKS

The standard advice is: to stay within the recommended limits and to avoid drinking on an empty stomach (risk of significant hypoglycaemia) or as a substitute for a meal. In type 2 diabetics, drinking two to three glasses of wine (or the equivalent quantity of beer) may produce an insignificant drop in blood glucose, but does not increase the risk of hypoglycaemia (Christiansen et al 1996). Alcohol is potentially a major energy source, but it can contribute to elevated blood pressure and serum triglycerides.

OTHER CIRCUMSTANCES

Older adults

Older diabetics are at risk of undernutrition, which should be considered when evaluating involuntary weight loss and should be avoided when implementing a weight-loss diet.

Hypertension

There are a number of dietary modifications that can contribute to lowering blood pressure:

- *Weight loss* in the overweight. A loss of 1 kg body weight produces a fall of 1 mmHg in mean arterial pressure.

- *Salt restriction*. The ADA's Expert Consensus recommends that the maximum daily intake of sodium should be 2400 mg (100 mmol), or 6000 mg of salt (sodium chloride) (ADA 2003). Reducing the daily intake from 12 g to 6 g can produce a fall in blood pressure of 5/2–3 mmHg. Salt restriction can potentiate the blood pressure-lowering effect of some agents in type 2 diabetics. However, since most commercial cereal and bread products contain 1% salt by weight, consuming these products increases the intake of both starchy carbohydrate and salt. It may be preferable to eat unsalted cereals and to replace some cereal foods with fruit and vegetables.
- *Reduce alcohol consumption*.

The American Dietary Approaches to Stop Hypertension (DASH) is an eating plan that advises hypertensive individuals to consume a diet rich in fruit, vegetables and low-fat dairy products with a reduced content of saturated and total fat. Those who follow this diet combined with sodium restriction can expect to their lower systolic blood pressure by 8 to 14 mmHg (Sacks et al 2001). The eating plan can be downloaded off the internet.

Although there appears to be an inverse relationship between blood pressure levels and the consumption of potassium (found in fruit and vegetables), magnesium and calcium, the 2004 BHS guidelines do *not* recommend supplementation of these minerals.

Different ethnic groups

The professional needs to tailor the advice given within the bounds of what is acceptable, attractive and realistic. Different Indo-Asian diets are suitable, provided that *total fat intake is reduced*. The manner in which food is prepared is important. While patients are encouraged to substitute olive oil for ghee in cooking, quantities should be measured and minimised.

REFERRAL TO DIETICIAN

Practice nurses and GPs are ideally placed to provide the basics of sound nutritional advice and should reinforce this as appropriate when reviews are undertaken. However, a referral to a qualified dietician for an individual dietary assessment is appropriate:

- when type 2 diabetes is diagnosed
- when insulin is started
- when other medical problems are present (e.g. obesity, hyperlipidaemia, renal impairment)
- when the glycated haemoglobin remains persistently raised
- if the patient fails to achieve or maintain optimal body weight.

PHYSICAL ACTIVITY AND EXERCISE

NSF ◀
1

DEFINITIONS

Physical activity can be defined as any skeletal muscle movement that expends energy above resting level.

Exercise is a type of physical activity that is carried out to enhance or maintain an aspect of fitness.

RATIONALE

A sedentary lifestyle is associated with an increased risk of coronary heart disease (CHD). Sedentary individuals are more likely to be obese and have adverse lipid profiles. In one study that recruited diabetic women, those undertaking less than 1 hour per week or no physical activity doubled their risk of having a cardiovascular event, compared to those undertaking at least 7 hours per week of physical activity (Hu et al 2001). Another study that recruited diabetic men found that "low" baseline cardio-respiratory fitness nearly trebled overall mortality compared with "moderate" or "high" fitness, and overall mortality nearly doubled in those reporting no recreational exercise in the previous 3 months, compared to those reporting any recreational physical activity in the same period (Wei et al 2000).

There is no current evidence to demonstrate a direct relationship between levels of physical activity and the development of the macrovascular and microvascular complications of diabetes. The arguments in favour of increased physical activity are based upon extrapolation from the effect of exercise on glycaemia. A recent report by the Chief Medical Officer distinguishes between the preventive effects (which appear to be strong) and the therapeutic effects of physical activity in type 2 diabetics (Department of Health 2004). The key message is that "the correct type of exercise is good".

Exercise has both short- and long-term benefits in type 2 patients (see Table 2.2). Exercise can be an effective way to reduce the risk of cardiovascular disease (CVD) (Pierce 1999): an appropriate level of physical activity, particularly in conjunction with diet, can improve cardiovascular risk factors, such as blood pressure, weight and lipids. A Cochrane meta-analysis of 14 RCTs "showed that exercise … improves glycaemic control and reduces visceral adipose tissue and plasma triglycerides, but not plasma cholesterol, … even without weight loss" (Thomas et al 2006).

TARGETS

Most diabetics should seek to be more physically active. The type and level of physical activity undertaken on a regular basis should be appropriate and enjoyable to the individual, and should promote endurance, muscle strength and flexibility – reducing cardiovascular risk.

Published guidelines give criteria for the intensity, type, frequency and duration of physical activity that should be fulfilled in an exercise programme for diabetics. Some of the more important guidelines are summarised in Table 2.3.

EVALUATION PRIOR TO UNDERTAKING AN EXERCISE PROGRAMME

Evaluation may be difficult. As well as eliciting details about the frequency, duration, type and intensity of physical activity, the professional should consider the attitude of the patient towards exercise, and social and cultural factors.

TABLE 2.2 The benefits of exercise for type 2 patients (ADA 1995, Buckley et al 1999)

Metabolic:

Reduced short-term insulin resistance; long-term effect has yet to be established
Increased peripheral glucose uptake
Less atherogenic profile (decreased triglycerides and LDL cholesterol with a beneficial increase in HDL cholesterol)
There is still no clear consensus on whether physical training results in improved fibrinolytic activity, which is impaired in type 2 diabetics

Reduces hypertension, particularly when hyperinsulinaemia is present

Helps to maintain muscle mass and promote preferentially the loss of adipose tissue, which may reduce the fall in metabolic rate during slimming and accelerate long-term weight loss

Favours weight loss by increasing energy expenditure (although an ageing overweight type 2 diabetic will be hard pressed to maintain the necessary daily level of exercise), in combination with a "slimming" diet

Prevention: physical activity undertaken in early adult life protects against the subsequent development of type 2 diabetes in middle-aged men and women (Ha & Lean 1997) and in patients with impaired glucose tolerance (Tuomilehto et al 2001)

Prior to beginning an exercise programme, a diabetic needs to be assessed for the following:

- The presence of *coronary artery disease* (or of several cardiovascular risk factors) requires a proper evaluation of the ischaemic response to increased levels of physical activity and of any propensity to arrhythmia during exercise.
- The presence of *peripheral neuropathy* may result in loss of protective sensation in the feet. Repetitive weight-bearing exercises (such as treadmill, jogging and step exercises) can be traumatic to insensitive feet and can ultimately risk ulceration. Non-weight-bearing exercises, such as swimming, bicycling, arm and chair exercises, avoid this risk. Proper footwear and adequate foot care are always necessary, whatever form of exercise is undertaken.
- The presence of *autonomic neuropathy* may limit an individual's capacity for physical activity and increase the risk of a sudden adverse cardiovascular event. Cardiac autonomic neuropathy (CAN) may be suggested by the presence of other disturbances in the autonomic nervous system (affecting skin, pupils, gastrointestinal and/or genitourinary systems), by a resting tachycardia (resting pulse greater than 100 beats per minute), or by orthostasis (a drop in systolic blood pressure of greater than 20 mmHg when standing).
- Those with *active retinopathy*, in particular *proliferative*, must avoid activities (such as vigorous aerobic or resistance exercise) that increase systolic blood pressure, involve Valsalva manoeuvres or are jarring, since these types of exercise can increase substantially the risk of retinal detachment (ADA 1995).

TABLE 2.3 Recommended criteria for exercise programmes

Parameter	Recommedations			
	Chief Medical Officer (DoH 2004) Not specifically for diabetics	NICE (NICE 2006b)	ADA (ADA 2007)	American College of Sports Medicine (Beers & Berkow 1999)
Frequency (times per week)	5 or more	5 or more	Aerobic: At least 3 ("with no more than 2 consecutive days without physical activity") Resistance: 3 times per week	3 to 5 (2 for resistive strength training)
Intensity	"Moderate"	"Moderate"	Moderate: 50 to 70% of maximum heart rate (= 220 − age in years) or Vigorous: >70% of maximum heart rate	Either to 60–90% of maximum heart rate (= 220 − age in years) or to a heart rate at 50–85% of maximum O_2 uptake
Duration	30 minutes for general health benefit or 45 to 60 minutes to prevent obesity	30 minutes	Aerobic: At least 150 minutes (per week) of moderate exercise or At least 90 minutes (per week) of vigorous exercise	20–60 minutes of continuous aerobic activity, depending upon intensity
Type and methods	"Brisk walking, cycling, and swimming"	From: 1. Tailored physical activity programme 2. Pedometers 3. Community-based walking or cycling programme	Aerobic plus resistance: Targeting all major muscle groups (8 to 10 repetitions at a weight that cannot be lifted more than 8 to 10 times) Energy expenditure: modulate to achieve 700 to 2000 calories per week	Rhythmic and aerobic, using large muscle groups (For resistive strength training: One set of 8–12 repetitions of 8–10 exercises Condition the major muscle groups)

- If peripheral arterial pulses are absent, then *peripheral arterial disease* may be present; this can be assessed by carrying out Doppler pressures (referral to a vascular surgeon).
- Although increased physical activity can increase urinary protein excretion, there is no evidence that vigorous exercise has an adverse effect on *diabetic nephropathy*. There are no specific exercise restrictions for people with diabetic kidney disease.

INTERVENTIONS

The recommendations of different authoritative bodies list several criteria that a suitable exercise programme for patients with diabetes should fulfil, summarised in Table 2.3. Most recommend that exercise should be:

- Aerobic plus (in the absence of contra-indications) resistance
- Undertaken at least three times per week
- At least 150 minutes total duration per week
- Of moderate intensity (50 to 70% of maximum heart rate).

NICE has published guidance on brief interventions that professionals can use to advise inactive individuals to increase levels of physical activity. NICE's recommendations include that health-care professionals should:

- Identify inactive adults, and advise them to aim to undertake 30 minutes of moderate activity on 5 or more days of the week.
- Provide written advice with agreed goals that takes into account "an individual's needs, preferences and circumstances".
- Follow up these individuals "at appropriate intervals over a 3 to 6 month period" (NICE 2006b).

NICE's options for increased physical activity include approved exercise referral schemes, use of pedometers, and walking and cycling schemes. However, it does admit that there is "insufficient evidence to recommend the use of pedometers and walking and cycling schemes to promote physical activity, other than as part of research studies where effectiveness can be evaluated" (NICE 2006b).

The "ideal" may not be desirable or realistic for all diabetics. In any exercise programme, essential precautions are the inclusion of proper warm up and cooling down, suitable foot care, and adequate hydration and metabolic control (Ruderman et al 2002).

Both attitude to change and social and/or cultural factors need to be considered before undertaking any exercise programme. The goals set determine the balance, duration, intensity and methods of exercise to undertake after the evaluation. The ideal exercise programme combines aerobic (e.g. walking, running, cycling, dancing, swimming, skipping) and anaerobic (e.g. resistive strength training of major muscle groups) activities. The latter have been shown to reduce vascular risk by decreasing resting blood pressure, increasing HDL cholesterol and decreasing insulin resistance.

There are a number of exercise schemes that may be accessible and suitable for diabetics:

1. *Exercise prescription schemes* offer supervised low-cost exercise for those unwilling and/or unable to visit a gym. They are run as a collaboration between local medical services and sports facilities, and GP practices refer patients via a "prescription".
2. *Local sports centres* may offer special sessions for over 50s, disabled people and pregnant women.
3. *Specialist rehabilitation schemes* may be run by specialist services and include exercise and education for patients with specific conditions (e.g. post-MI).

Health-care professionals should take great care to ensure that any exercise programme is safe, appropriate to patients' general physical condition, suitable to their lifestyle and goals, and enjoyable. It is important that exercise includes proper warm-up and cool-down periods; this should also reduce the risk of injury.

Further information about Quality Assurance for exercise programmes is on the Department of Health's website (*http://www.dh.gov.uk*). An American perspective is given in the Surgeon General's report on Physical Activity and Health (US Department of Health 1996).

Table 2.4 gives guidance about maintaining glycaemic control during exercise.

TABLE 2.4 Guidelines for a diabetic's optimal glycaemic response to exercise

Metabolic control before exercise

Avoid exercise if fasting glucose levels are > 14 mmol/l with ketosis present, and use caution if glucose levels are > 17 mmol/l without ketosis present
Ingest added carbohydrate if glucose levels are < 5.5 mmol/l

Blood glucose monitoring before and after exercise

Identify when changes in insulin or food intake are required
Learn the glycaemic response to different exercise situations

Food intake

Consume added carbohydrate as needed to avoid hypoglycaemia
Carbohydrate should be readily available during and after exercise

Hypoglycaemia

Beware that sulphonylureas and insulin may cause hypoglycaemia during exercise; if exercise is anticipated, doses may need to be reduced (by up to 65% of insulin for vigorous exercise up to 45 minutes)
Avoid injecting insulin into exercising areas, which increases its absorption and the risk of hypoglycaemia

SMOKING

RATIONALE

Half of all smokers die as a result of a smoking-related ailment. Smoking is a major aetiological factor not only for cardiovascular disease and peripheral vascular disease, but also for lung cancer and respiratory conditions. There is a dose correlation between CHD risk and the number of cigarettes smoked daily.

The UKPDS identified smoking as a risk factor for coronary artery disease in type 2 diabetics (Turner 1998). Smoking also promotes the development of microvascular complications of diabetes (retinopathy, nephropathy and foot disease).

Cigarette smoking increases cardiovascular risk by:

- Elevating low-density lipoprotein (LDL) and lowering high-density lipoprotein (HDL) cholesterol levels
- Raising blood carbon monoxide (producing endothelial hypoxia)
- Promoting vasoconstriction of arteries already narrowed by arteriosclerosis
- Increasing platelet reactivity that may lead to platelet thrombus formation
- Increasing plasma fibrinogen concentration, resulting in greater blood viscosity.

Although the main benefits of smoking cessation are the reduction of all-cause mortality and the development of CVD (CHD, stroke and especially PVD; Macleod 1994), there is evidence now emerging that patients with diabetes may be able to reduce their risk of developing some diabetes complications, such as nephropathy and neuropathy by giving up smoking.

It is a source of optimism that the proportion of the English population that smokes has declined. The latest Health Survey for England (NHS Health and Social Care Information Centre 2004) found that:

- The proportion of men currently smoking declined from 28% in 1993 to 22% in 2004.
- The proportion of women current smoking declined from 26% in 1993 to 23% in 2004.
- The proportion of diabetics who smoke is the same as non-diabetics (Wingard et al 2002).

AIMS

The main aim is to enable and maintain the cessation of smoking.

However, since smoking is a behaviour that is ultimately under the patient's control, any "target" set must be negotiated and agreed with the patient. Smoking cessation may not be desired by or achievable in some patients: the patient and clinician may have to settle for minimising the extent of the patient's smoking. Ex-smokers should be discouraged from re-starting smoking.

ASSESSMENT

The patient should be asked:

- What is smoked
- The current quantities
- Any recent changes in behaviour.

If the patient is an ex-smoker, it may be helpful to enquire about any problems encountered and the patient's attitude to his future as a non-smoker.

If the patient is a current smoker, it is also useful to ascertain:

- The patient's attitude to smoking cessation
- Details and success of previous attempts to stop smoking
- What barriers are present to prevent the patient from stopping
- Likely future plans to try to stop smoking.

In patients who are currently or are suspected of smoking, devices can be acquired to check blood levels of carbon monoxide.

The above information may inform the professional's choice of strategies to use that are mostly likely to promote smoking cessation. Any information elicited should be documented in the clinical records, including if a patient is reluctant to consider change or if any positive encouragement was given to an ex-smoker (NICE 2006a).

It is important for the professional to identify any patient who smokes and may be on the verge of changing behaviour: taking such an opportunity to provide immediate and effective support, using one or more of the interventions discussed below, may achieve a higher rate of success in smoking cessation.

INTERVENTIONS

If the patient is a non-smoker, the clinician may wish to offer positive encouragement for the patient to continue this behaviour, possibly re-iterating the benefits of smoking and the disadvantages of resuming.

Following its White Paper *Smoking Kills* in 1998, the Government's tobacco programme has included the following:

- A comprehensive NHS Stop Smoking Service set up in 1999. This had a budget of £112 000 000 for the two financial years 2006/2007 and 2007/2008 (DoH Tobacco Policy online).
- High-profile public health and media campaigns to highlight the dangers of smoking.
- Funding of initiatives such as counselling services, a helpline (NHS Smoking Helpline).
- Regulations for reducing tobacco promotion and advertising, and increases in tobacco duties.
- Legislation for the banning of smoking in enclosed public places was passed in 2006 for implementation in the summer of 2007.
- The availability on the NHS of the smoking cessation aids NRT and bupropion.

A variety of the available strategies to promote smoking cessation are effective (Lancaster et al 2000). In 2002 NICE recommended that both bupropion and nicotine replacement therapy should be funded by the NHS (NICE Appraisal Committee 2002).

A patient unwilling to consider the benefits of or how to initiate any action to make change is extremely unlikely to respond to any intervention. In such circumstances, all the professional can do is to briefly emphasise the positive health and social benefits of becoming a nonsmoker while underlining the considerable risks of remaining a smoker. Handled sensitively, "the door is left open" and, possibly, a useful idea is planted. In a cross-sectional household survey, nearly half of those who had quit smoking did so as an unplanned attempt: once the decision was made to quit, immediate action was taken without planning (West & Sohal 2006). Professionals need to recognise a patient's level of motivation in order to target their interventions at those most likely to respond.

Since smoking is a behaviour owned by the individual who does it, any change to this behaviour is also owned by the same individual. Any intervention by a health-care professional needs to respect this concept and be directed at "empowering" the patient to make and implement positive and beneficial choices.

Advice

Brief focused interventions consisting of advice given by health professionals can achieve smoking cessation rates of 2% (University of York 1998) and may be the "key" to persuading more smokers to stop (West 2005). NICE has provided guidance on brief interventions by professionals to promote smoking cessation, recommending that these may take 5 to 10 minutes and should include one or more of the following:

- Providing simple advice to stop
- Evaluating the patient's commitment to quit
- Offering pharmacotherapy and/or behavioural support
- Providing self-help material and making a referral for more intensive support, such as the NHS Stop Smoking Services.

NICE calculated that if professionals carried out the above, the smoking cessation rate could increase to 4.3% (NICE 2006).

There is evidence that counselling over the telephone is effective without face-to-face contact (Zhu et al 1996). When more "intensive" telephone counselling (using behavioural methods) is combined with NRT, smoking cessation rates are significantly higher (An et al 2006).

NICE guidance for prescribing smoking cessation aids

In its 2002 technology appraisal, NICE recommended that:

- NRT or bupropion should only be prescribed to smokers who commit to a target stop date.
- Neither NRT nor bupropion should be prescribed to smokers under the age of 18 years.
- NRT and bupropion should not be prescribed in combination.

- The initial prescription of NRT should provide sufficient quantities to last for 2 weeks after the target stop date. The initial prescription of bupropion should be sufficient to last for 3–4 weeks after the target stop date.
- Second prescriptions for NRT and bupropion should only be given to those who have demonstrated that their attempt to quit is being sustained.
- If an attempt to stop smoking is unsuccessful, the NHS should not normally fund a further attempt with NRT or bupropion within 6 months.

Smoking cessation clinics

As part of the tobacco campaign, smoking cessation clinics have been set up throughout the NHS in increasing numbers. These clinics are directly accessible to patients and are run by trained counsellors. They can provide starter courses of smoking cessation aids (such as NRT and bupropion). Many practices are also running their own smoking cessation programmes. With appropriate training and organisational support, practice nurses are ideally placed to run these clinics. Smoking cessation clinics are more effective than brief advice or usual care in motivated "quitters".

Nicotine replacement therapy (NRT)

The available formulations of NRT include transdermal patches, chewing gum, inhalation or nasal spray for physical withdrawal symptoms, e.g. the first cigarette before breakfast (see BNF section 4.10 for further details). All forms are effective and are available either over the counter or on an NHS prescription. The dose depends upon the number of cigarettes smoked per day.

There are over 50 RCTs comparing NRT against placebo in the Cochrane database. A Cochrane review found all of the commercially available forms of NRT to be effective as part of a strategy to promote smoking cessation. Compared to placebo, NRT doubled quit rates after 1 year in motivated patients. NRT effectiveness appears to be largely independent of the intensity of additional support provided to the smoker (Silagy et al 2004).

NRT is quite safe, but NICE recommends caution in patients with cardiovascular disease, hyperthyroidism, severe renal or hepatic impairment and peptic ulcer, as well as diabetes (although the dangers of continuing to smoke usually far outweigh the potential side effects of NRT). Some formulations of NRT are contra-indicated in pregnancy.

Antidepressants

The antidepressants *bupropion* (Zyban – see BNF section 4.10) and *nortriptyline* have increased smoking cessation rates in a small number of trials. Only some antidepressants aid smoking cessation independently of the presence of depressive symptoms, suggesting that their mode of action is not linked to their therapeutic antidepressant effect (Hughes et al 2004). Patients in these trials were offered also behavioural support; these drugs should be prescribed within a structured counselling programme (Lancaster et al 2000).

Bupropion is available currently on NHS prescription for smoking cessation. The main adverse events associated with bupropion are seizures, which occur in about 1 in 1000 patients. In addition, it is also recommended that patients prescribed bupropion should have their blood pressure monitored, as rises have been reported even in normotensive individuals.

Varenicline

This is a new class of medication that acts centrally (targeting the α4β2 nicotinic receptor), reducing both the pleasurable effect associated with nicotine and withdrawal side effects. The manufacturer claims superior quit rates to bupropion at 12 weeks, no known drug interactions and good tolerability (nausea is the commonest side effect). Dosage should be adjusted in "moderate to severe" renal impairment. It should be started one to two weeks before the target stop date and is a twelve week course. Like other smoking cessation products, prescribing varenicline should be combined with appropriate counselling and support. In May 2007, NICE recommended varenicline as an option for adult smokers who have expressed a desire to quit.

Other methods of smoking cessation

Other methods that have been used for smoking cessation are considered either ineffective (anxiolytics and lobeline), of uncertain benefit (acupuncture, aversion therapy, hypnotherapy), or limited by side effects (*clonidine*). It is possible that the cannabinoid receptor antagonist, *rimonabant* (discussed in Chapter 4), may have potential in aiding smoking cessation.

ALCOHOL

RATIONALE

There is an inverse relationship between alcohol consumption and the risk of CHD mortality (Valmadrid et al 1999, Ajani et al 2000); however, moderate alcohol consumption may offer some protection against stroke (Sacco et al 1999). There are no data available on alcohol consumption and the risk of developing peripheral vascular disease (PVD). There is no evidence that alcohol is a risk factor for the development of diabetic neuropathy.

Alcoholic cardiomyopathy may develop after 10 years of heavy alcohol abuse, due to a direct toxic effect of alcohol upon cardiac muscle. Alcohol abuse is also associated with thiamine deficiency, which can contribute to the development of cardiomyopathy. Alcohol consumption can affect levels of blood pressure, blood glucose and serum triglycerides.

Regular excessive alcohol consumption can also have serious adverse effects upon the psychological well-being of the patient and others, often leading to depression and, in extreme cases, to social chaos.

ASSESSMENT

Alcohol consumption is measured in units, with 1 unit equating to:

- 9 g ethanol
- 1 spirits measure
- 1 glass wine
- ½ pint beer.

A bottle of spirits usually contains 26 to 28 units.

History

A sensible starting point is to ask the patient. However, denial is a frequent feature of alcoholism; thus, some patients may not be entirely forthcoming about their alcohol consumption and other members of the household or friends may prove more informative.

If there is suspicion that the patient may be drinking excessively, then a useful screening test to use is the CAGE questionnaire:

- Have you ever felt you should **c**ut down on your drinking?
- Have you ever felt **a**nnoyed at others' concerns about your drinking?
- Have you ever felt **g**uilty about drinking?
- Have you ever had alcohol as an **e**ye-opener in the morning?

Two or more positive answers suggest an alcohol problem exists.

Examination

Abnormal physical signs may not always be present, but clinicians should look for signs of liver damage, slurred speech, sweating, tremor, and the smell of alcohol, particularly in dependent drinkers.

Investigations

Blood tests may be useful for screening excessive alcohol consumption: a raised mean corpuscular volume (MCV) on the blood count and/or raised gamma-GT on the liver function test.

TARGETS

Unlike smoking, moderate alcohol consumption on a regular basis, but not in binges, is not harmful. Risk is a continuum and higher limits are controversial. "Low-risk" drinking is less than 21 units per week in men and 14 units per week in women. Diabetics are advised to avoid drinking more than 3 units of alcohol in one session.

REDUCING ALCOHOL CONSUMPTION

Reducing alcohol consumption, particularly when it is far above the recognised safe upper limit, is often very challenging and its success depends upon a patient's willingness and commitment to change. The principles are the same for all patients, both non-diabetic and diabetic.

In non-dependent drinkers, particularly those receptive to change, about one-quarter may reduce their drinking following brief GP interventions: these include providing information about safe limits and the harm of excess, and agreeing target consumption and review. Since alcohol-dependent drinkers are likely to suffer withdrawal symptoms (e.g. anxiety, fits, delirium tremens) if they reduce their alcohol consumption, detoxification is required. Although possible in the community, the presence of severe physical, psychological and/or social problems or previous complicated withdrawals, requires detoxification to be undertaken as an inpatient. Such patients should be referred early to the community alcohol team.

In these complex situations, primary care can still play a useful role by:

- Evaluating willingness and barriers to change, and any target organ damage
- Providing information
- Prescribing vitamins (especially thiamine) during withdrawal
- Liaising with other services
- Supporting the patient's family.

Sources of support and advice for patients include:

- *Drinkline* (government-sponsored helpline): telephone 0800 9178282
- *Alcohol Concern* online: *http://www.alcoholconcern.org.uk*
- *Alcoholics Anonymous*: telephone 0845 7697555; online: *http://www.alcoholics-anonymous.org.uk* (also links to section for professionals).

PATIENT EDUCATION AND LIFESTYLE MODIFICATION

NSF ◀
3

A patient with type 2 diabetes "owns" his disease and plays a crucial role in his own glycaemic control, current and future well-being and prevention of complications. Diabetes education has shifted from a didactic approach, centred on imparting information, to a skill-based approach centred on helping diabetics to make informed appropriate self-management choices. The latter approach is more likely to change "risky" behaviour and to improve lifestyle.

Diabetes education begins with diagnosis. Each subsequent professional encounter with the patient should be regarded as an opportunity for education. Primary care professionals trained to take a "patient-centred" approach when addressing lifestyle are more likely than those in secondary care to improve the patient's satisfaction and knowledge (Kinmouth et al 1998). Other (non-medical) factors may affect a patient's current and future behaviour. Until these issues are addressed, changes and improved care will be delayed or less likely to result.

GENERAL PRINCIPLES OF THE PROCESS OF HEALTH EDUCATION

- *Good communication* is essential, however the health education is delivered. There is a clear correlation between effective doctor–patient communication and improved patient health outcomes (Stewart 1995). Some thought needs to be given as to how to understand and reach out to diabetics who do not speak English, such as elderly Indo-Asians. Access to an interpreter and appropriate written and/or electronic material is helpful.
- The patient's *needs are identified and addressed*. The content of any health education package should be geared to the time of and the need for its use.
- Where appropriate, the patient's *willingness and barriers to change are identified*.
- The patient and the team *agree the aims of care* and the methods used to achieve these aims. These need to be realistic, respect the patient's autonomy, increase the patient's freedom of action, and have perceived and sustained benefit. Failure to agree will not change an unhealthy lifestyle.

- Advice given is *based upon the evidence* and *appropriate* to the patient's psychological and social circumstances.
- A clear *explanation about the importance and rationale* of any advice or intervention is provided.
- *Expectations* of performance, by both the patient and/or professional, are *realistic*. Otherwise, disappointment is more likely, and the perceived failure is likely to result in poor concordance.
- All the involved professionals give *consistent advice* (stay "on message").
- *Prepare the patient for changes* as the need arises.

STRUCTURES AND PROCESSES FOR THE DELIVERY OF DIABETES EDUCATION

Background

NICE published a technology appraisal in 2003 of patient education models for diabetes. NICE defined structured education as "a planned and graded programme that is comprehensive in scope, flexible in content, responsive to an individual's clinical and psychological needs, and adaptable to his or her educational and cultural background" (NICE 2003). Following this, a joint Diabetes UK and the Department of Health Patient Education Working Group published a report in 2005 highlighting best practice for a structured educational programme that can fulfil the requirements in the NICE definition (DoH, Diabetes UK 2005).

Structured educational programmes

The working group agreed that the key critria for a structured educational programme could be divided into five main areas:

1. The *philosophy* of the programme should be that it is evidence-based, flexible to the individual's needs, and supportive of self-management, with specific learning objectives.
2. The *curriculum* needs to be structured, person-centred, evidence-based, resource-effective and flexible.
3. *Educators* need to be properly *trained*.
4. A *Quality Assurance* programme needs to be in place, with competent independent assessment.
5. The *outcomes* from the programme need to be *audited*.

There are currently two national group education programmes in the UK for adults with diabetes that fulfil the above criteria:

1. **DAFNE** (Dose Adjustment For Normal Eating) is a skills-based programme taught over 5 days in a hospital outpatients (following rigorous research) to groups of adults with *type 1* diabetes, aimed at teaching the patient how to adjust insulin to suit his free choice of food, rather than working his life around the dose of insulin. The NICE technology appraisal concluded that DAFNE is cost-effective. As of June 2006, there were 37 trained DAFNE centres throughout the UK and Ireland that have trained over 4000 patients. More information can be found on the DAFNE website: *http://www.dafne.uk.com/*

2. **DESMOND** (Diabetes Education for Self-Management: Ongoing and Newly Diagnosed) is for adults newly diagnosed with *type 2* diabetes and has already generated considerable interest. DESMOND was piloted in 2004, followed by an RCT (due to report). It is now being rolled out nationally. The commitment from the patient is to attend two 3-hour sessions (on the same day or within a fortnight), led by a trained educator, of a structured group (up to 10) education programme, aimed at supporting the patient to become more expert about and, thus, better able to self-manage his diabetes. Follow-up questionnaires are sent out every 12 months after the course. More information can be found on the project website: *www.desmond-project.org.uk.*

Local adult education programmes are also being developed. A successful example is the Diabetes X-PERT Programme; a structured group education programme based upon the theories of empowerment and discovery learning. More information can be found on the programme's website: *www.xpert-diabetes.org.uk.*

Specific topics of health education suitable for diabetics

The curriculum of health education topics for a patient with diabetes is large, in depth, range and the number of techniques to be used. In broad terms, these can be placed under the following headings:

- Lifestyle: diet and alcohol consumption, smoking and physical activity
- Glycaemic control: self-monitoring and administration of therapy (e.g. insulin)
- Reduction of cardiovascular risk: weight management, blood pressure, lipids
- Complications: foot care
- Practical issues: prescriptions, follow-up, employment, driving, travel.

Types of educational interventions

Reviews of the evidence on the effectiveness of different interventions on modifying the lifestyle of diabetics have been carried out by SIGN (SIGN 2001), the University of Sheffield (McIntosh et al 2002), and the NICE technology appraisal (NICE 2003). NICE concluded that there was insufficient evidence to recommend a specific type of education or to provide guidance on the settings for and frequency of sessions. There are still substantial gaps, but there is a considerable volume of on-going research, and it is hoped that the picture should become progressively clearer.

NICE's suggestions for the principles of good practice include:

- Education should reflect adult learning principles
- Preference for group work using an appropriately trained multidisciplinary team
- Access to the broadest selection of people
- Use of a variety of suitable and patient-centred techniques.

The different educational methods include:

- Didactic-based approach – little interaction or evidence of benefit.
- Behaviour-modification approach – uses a broad range of strategies, focussing

mostly on diet and exercise. It helps weight reduction, but there is less evidence for improvements in glycaemic control and knowledge.

- Telephone-delivered education – used increasingly for queries and to adjust the management of on-going problems, reducing the pressure on overstretched appointment systems. The advantages may be greater flexibility and convenience for both patient and professional, but an examination or any nonverbal evaluation is not possible.

- Group-management approach – limited evidence of benefit and requires organisation.

- Skills demonstration – delivered by either a practice member or an invited "resource". It appears to be effective, although further research is needed.

- Computer-assisted learning – limited evidence suggests that they improve knowledge. Such packages are not yet freely available in primary care. GP computer software has access to patient information systems, from which information leaflets can be printed off. Also, numerous websites provide high-quality information (see Appendix 4), but these are not interactive and are unlikely to change behaviour.

- Combination of teaching methods – includes group and individual education, counselling, videotapes, "empowerment" strategies, peer support and biofeedback-relaxation training. Some of these components are not easily available in primary care, but those involved in professional education already use a "multi-faceted" approach that can be applied to patient education.

- Patient activation-involvement approach – uses a variety of strategies, and aims to encourage patients to become more involved in their care, particularly in decision-making. Evidence for its benefits in diabetic health education is limited to possible improvements in HbA1c and patient's knowledge. It is not really a method, more an aim.

A PSYCHOLOGICAL APPROACH TO HEALTH EDUCATION CONSULTATIONS

A personal view

Many GPs and practice nurses lack both the time and skills to provide effective health education for their patients, although providing suitable advice may be an essential component of disease management. Most professionals attempt to provide short bursts of "health education" in consultations that deal with chronic disease. Over a long period the total time devoted to such interventions is considerable. Is this time well spent? Occasionally, a professional has "miraculously" changed a patient's behaviour with a single piece of appropriate advice. Increasing the "success rate" would benefit patients and increase professionals' job satisfaction.

Every professional can easily create a list of the "usual suspects", regular consulters whose chronic problems are caused or exacerbated by their poor lifestyle, and who remain impervious to any suggestions for modifying their behaviour, while simultaneously and eternally expecting the professional to provide the nonexistent "miracle cure". Improving lifestyle in these individuals is a huge challenge.

Patients often know more than is credited about their disease and other health matters. The priority of health education is more often to facilitate behavioural change than to simply "spoon feed" information. This requires an approach that is not didactic, but that does draw upon the working methods of educationalists and psychologists.

It is useful to draw upon four overlapping concepts in a simplistic way to enhance the effectiveness of educational interventions within the consultation:

- Effective consultation technique
- The educational triangle
- The model of change
- Cognitive behaviour therapy.

Effective consultation technique

Effective consultation behaviours in all patient contacts, without ignoring clinical issues, are more likely to facilitate changes in a patient's behaviour. A review published in the BMJ provides a helpful list of concepts and techniques (Gask & Usherwood 2002), but there is a wealth of excellent literature (Launer 2002, Pendleton et al 2003).

"Successful" consultations are more likely to result if:

- A constructive relationship is built
- The professional's skills are deployed effectively to define problems and to generate potential solutions
- Emotional and social factors also are considered in both diagnosis and management
- The patient's agenda is elicited and addressed
- The patient is involved appropriately in any decision-making process and management plan. This has been shown to achieve better blood glucose and blood pressure control (Kaplan et al 1989).

One of the authors (SL) has developed his own consultation model that aims to clarify behaviours within consultations more likely to produce beneficial outcomes (see Figure 2.1).

Educational triangle

The triad of "aims, methods and assessment" can also be applied to health education:

1. **Aims** address any combination of knowledge, skill or attitude "needs", as agreed by the learner and the provider.
2. **Methods** may involve a range of activities from one-on-one to groups, printed and video literature and electronic resources.
3. **Assessment** is "formative" and requires repeating regularly, so as to provide the information needed to revise and prioritise the patient's educational needs.

Models of change
Trans-theoretical model of change

In the 1980s the "trans-theoretical model of change" for addiction behaviours was published (Prochaska & DiClemente 1992). Many professionals began to recognise

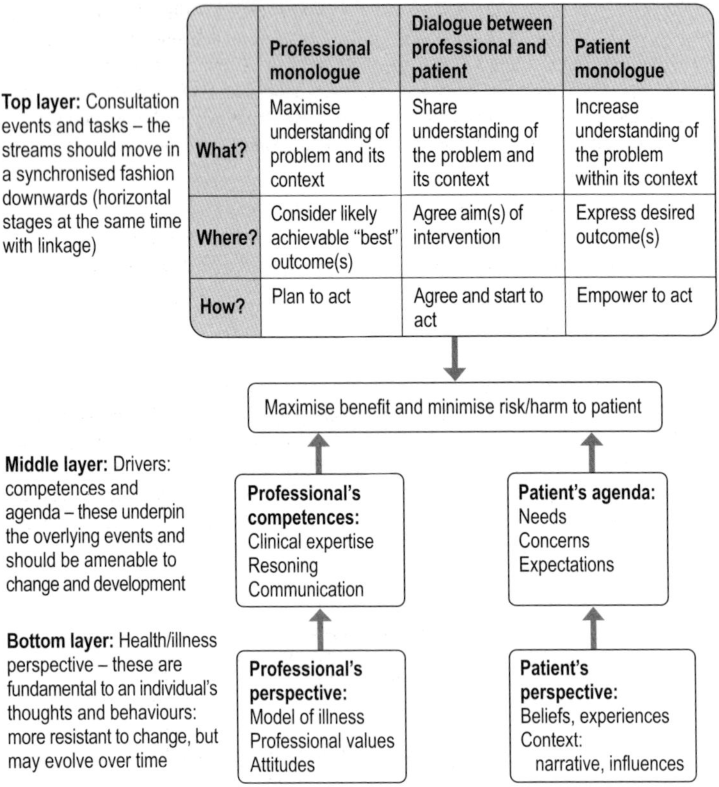

Top layer: Consultation events and tasks – the streams should move in a synchronised fashion downwards (horizontal stages at the same time with linkage)

		Professional monologue	Dialogue between professional and patient	Patient monologue
	What?	Maximise understanding of problem and its context	Share understanding of the problem and its context	Increase understanding of the problem within its context
	Where?	Consider likely achievable "best" outcome(s)	Agree aim(s) of intervention	Express desired outcome(s)
	How?	Plan to act	Agree and start to act	Empower to act

Maximise benefit and minimise risk/harm to patient

Middle layer: Drivers: competences and agenda – these underpin the overlying events and should be amenable to change and development

Professional's competences:
Clinical expertise
Resoning
Communication

Patient's agenda:
Needs
Concerns
Expectations

Bottom layer: Health/illness perspective – these are fundamental to an individual's thoughts and behaviours: more resistant to change, but may evolve over time

Professional's perspective:
Model of illness
Professional values
Attitudes

Patient's perspective:
Beliefs, experiences
Context:
   narrative, influences

Fig. 2.1 Schematic representation of consultation model

that the model (summarised in Figure 2.2) could be applied to various health-related behaviours, such as smoking, alcohol consumption, diet and exercise. This model is particularly attractive because it recognises that different strategies are required to further change at each stage, and because it reflects the progress and relapse that occurs in real life.

A patient who is uninterested in change is at the *pre-contemplative* stage. A patient thinking about change (at the *contemplative* stage) can be helped through the sequential stages of *preparation*, *action* and *maintenance*, leading to safer or healthier behaviour. Relapse can occur but, if recognised, patients can be guided back to the preparation and action stages.

Various triggers may cause a patient to move from being unwilling to being prepared to think about change. This transformation may result from realising that an adverse event may be imminent or more likely, that the problem is connected to current behaviour, and that the benefits of change outweigh the risks and/or disadvantages. If a patient appears unwilling to change, then the professional may wish to use one or more of the following strategies to help the patient move from the pre-contemplation to contemplation:

- Emphasise the positive health and social benefits of change
- Focus upon the risks of maintaining a particular unhealthy aspect of lifestyle
- Help the patient to demolish or find a route around any barriers to change.

Whatever strategy is used, the professional is likely to be seeking to alter the patient's motivation at this point.

Model of change based upon the "catastrophe theory"

An alternative to the trans-theoretical model has been proposed recently. This is based on a branch of mathematics, where tensions develop in a system so that even small "triggers" can cause "catastrophic" changes. It is proposed "that beliefs, past experiences, and the current situation create varying levels of 'motivational tension', in the presence of which even quite small 'triggers' can lead to … renunciation." If a plan for *later* action is the result, then this "may signify a lower level of commitment" in the individual (West & Sohal 2006).

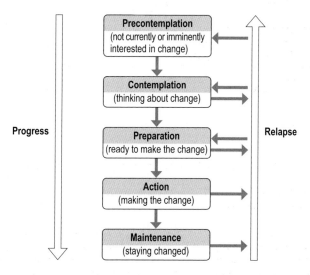

Fig. 2.2 The trans-theoretical model of change

West has incorporated this concept in a theory of motivation and how it can be applied to addictive behaviours (West 2006). He advises public health campaigns that seek to influence behaviours to focus on the "3 Ts":

1. Creating motivational **t**ension
2. **T**riggering action in those who are on the "cusp" of change in their "orientation" to an addictive behaviour, such as smoking
3. Immediate availability of **t**reatment to support attempts to change.

This theory recognises both the often sudden variability in an individual's motivations and the importance of a timely effective response by the professional to opportunities within a consultation that may be indicated by various cues given by the patient. The trans-theoretical and catastrophe theory models are not incompatible: the trans-theoretical model does not specify duration of time spent at any of its stages. An individual whose motivational tension is a high level, leading to renunciation and "unplanned" change, could be considered to have moved from pre-contemplation to action very rapidly through the contemplation and preparation stages in-between.

Cognitive behaviour therapy (CBT) and motivational approaches
Definitions
Cognitive behaviour therapy (CBT) refers to a group of psychological treatments that include behaviour therapy, behaviour modification and cognitive therapy in various combinations.

Behaviour approaches aim to change behaviour, both as a therapeutic aim in its own right, and to produce other symptomatic improvements.
Cognitive approaches explore how cognition mediates feelings and behaviour. Therapy aims to identify maladaptive thought patterns and to teach the patient to recognise and challenge these.

In practice, therapists combine both approaches (Richardson 1998).

Problem-solving
CBT has a wide range of established clinical applications, especially for mental health problems, such as depression, panic disorder and post-traumatic stress disorder (Enright 1997). There is now increasing interest in using CBT to modify other behaviours. The CBT process can be divided into three sequential steps (that can be undertaken over several encounters):

1. Baseline: "Where are you now?"
   Identify the patient's current state (behaviours, thoughts and feelings) with regard to his condition and well-being, prior to the process of goal setting. This information is important for developing rapport, for assisting change by starting the process of goal setting and for later evaluation.
2. Outcome: "Where do you want to get to?"

Ask the patient to define his goals and to consider his "picture of health"; the patient can be helped to explore the benefits of change, with attention to the expected gains (physical, psychological, cognitive). Goal identification also defines when the intervention is completed.

3. Process: "How are we going to get there?"

An agreed plan of action may include problem solving, graded task setting (small manageable goals that will generative greater self-confidence from success), visualisation, inter-personal "coaching", and other educational techniques. Both patient and professional will have clearly defined responsibilities in the implementation of the action plan.

Behavioural change can follow the above problem-solving steps. The Outcome stage of the CBT process equates to the "contemplative stage" of the trans-theoretical model.

Motivation

Motivation influences lifestyle and is owned by the individual. Levels of motivation can fluctuate: small triggers can produce sudden and dramatic changes. In order to better understand motivation so as to change it, the professional needs to be aware of the two main components of motivation:

1. **Importance**, made up of:
   - knowledge about gains and losses resulting from any particular behaviour
   - concern (balance between too little and too much) about that behaviour

   and

2. **Confidence**, made up of:
   - self-esteem
   - self-efficacy (belief in the individual's capability to act).

Structured information gathering by the professional will enable a greater understanding of the patient's current situation: the constructs of the patient's motivation (importance of current behaviour and his self-confidence) and an awareness of what outcomes might be feasible from behavioural change.

Simple questions can be asked to explore importance:

- "How do you feel now, on a scale of 1 to 10?"
- "On a scale of 1 to 10, how important is *xyz* to you?"
- "What would have to happen before you would seriously consider change?" and confidence:
- "How confident, on a scale of 1 to 10, do you feel about being able to change *xyz*?"
- "How can I help you to make that change?"
- "How successful have you been in previous attempts – what went wrong?"

If the status of a patient's motivational components are applied to the trans-theoretical model of change:

- at the pre-contemplation stage, the importance score will be low
- at the contemplation stage, the importance score will be high, but the confidence score may be low
- at the preparation stage, both importance and confidence scores need to be high.

To facilitate a patient's progress through the CBT process, the professional may wish to employ motivational interviewing techniques (summarised in Figure 2.3). Professionals can combine effective consulting techniques with motivational approaches and CBT. Those who seek to integrate these skills into their daily practice require training, practice and regular feedback.

Identifying and stimulating the patient's awareness of the need for change can use motivational "*linguistic patterns*" to emphasise the benefits of change; e.g. "As you begin eating more healthily and regularly, you will notice that your general well-being will improve. This will be because your blood sugar is becoming stable, and this, in turn, means that you will have more energy."

When the patient is ambivalent about the importance of change, it is useful to ask him to complete a grid, comparing the benefits and losses of change against those of no change (see Figure 2.4). Another strategy is to explore what would need to happen or alter to increase the importance of change for the patient. The patient should be able to express concerns about his current behaviour and the arguments for change, in order that his "decisional balance" is tipped towards action. This could also be seen as attempting to increase "motivational tension".

Where confidence is low, the professional needs to consider what "blocks" confidence; these may include:

- lack of knowledge and skills
- lack of support (from family, friends or professionals)
- past failures to change
- poor function (lack of alternative behaviours)
- psychological distress, such as anxiety, depression, low self-esteem.

The nature of the "block" will influence which strategy is used to try to dismantle it. It is sometimes helpful to ask a patient to recall previous strategies used to achieve success. The professional should have strong "interpersonal" skills and be able to negotiate with patients some specific plans with clear goals that require concrete actions in small steps, providing constructive feedback that develops a patient's ability to learn from "lapses".

The professional needs to be aware also of the effects of secondary gain, control and emotional expression within the patient's illness behaviour. Most people know what is good for them and how to achieve it. Just as smoking-cessation interventions are ineffective when the "benefits" to the patient of remaining a smoker are ignored, so too can some features be overlooked within the psychological management of

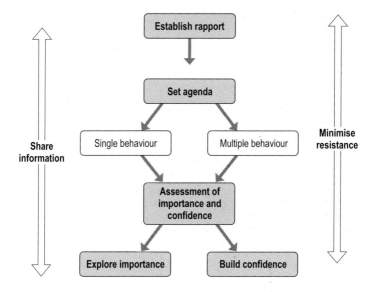

Fig. 2.3 The key tasks of motivational interviewing

	Benefits	Disadvantages
No change		
Change		

Fig. 2.4 Grid to help explore the benefits of change

physical conditions. An example is the patient who, after a row with his or her partner, sabotages some aspect of the diabetic programme (ignores diet, omits medication) to force the partner to take the roles of rescuer and consoler. This sabotage may be how a patient expresses anger, but it has negative health consequences. In contrast, healthy people under stress, who push themselves too far and risk adverse health, are not "saboteurs". The professional can uncover subconscious motives and challenge the patient, then help the patient take 'ownership' of his behaviour.

▶ KEY POINTS

- The important health educational messages are to eat sensibly, be more physically active, stop smoking, and to moderate alcohol intake.

- A healthy diet should provide essential nutrition, reduce cardiovascular risk and allow adaptation to metabolic problems.

- The main components of an exercise programme should include aerobic acitivity undertaken at least 3 times per week, of at least 150 minutes duration per week, and of moderate intensity (50 to 70% of maximum heart rate).

- Beyond simple advice, smokers should be offered help to quit using a variety of measures.

- Health education is more than imparting information; it should enable patients to make healthier choices.

- Busy professionals can employ effective techniques that may alter a patient's motivation. Behavioural rather than didactic approaches are more likely to succeed.

- Evidence for the benefits of various educational approaches remains limited.

GLYCAEMIC CONTROL

OVERVIEW

To achieve and maintain the targets (Table 3.1) of optimal glycaemic control can be difficult because of the progressive deterioration of pancreatic insulin secretion. Success is more likely if the patient, in collaboration with the professional and guided by monitoring of glycaemic control, masters the complex task of balancing the three key components of diet, physical activity and blood glucose-lowering medication dosage.

This chapter discusses self-monitoring and blood glucose-lowering medication. Diet and physical activity are discussed in Chapter 2.

MONITORING

Glycaemic control can be assessed in three complementary ways:

1. Glycosylated haemoglobin (or fructosamine)
2. Patient self-monitoring of either blood or urinary glucose
3. Patient symptoms.

TABLE 3.1 Targets for optimal glycaemic control

Target	Who monitors	Action
Avoiding hypoglycaemia	Patient	Recognises warning signs
		Balances regular meals, correct dose of therapy and physical activity
		Able to correct promptly
	Professional	Assesses needs and educates
Fasting blood glucose of 4 to 7 mmol/l	Patient	Able to do and interpret tests Adjusts therapy accordingly
	Professional	Assesses needs and educates
Glycated haemoglobin of less than 7.0%*	Patient	Understands significance of test result Adjusts therapy accordingly
	Professional	Repeats regularly
		Advises on appropriate therapy changes

*Individualised HbA1c targets should be set between 6.5 and 7.5%; the lower value is preferred for patients at significant risk of vascular complications, the higher may be more appropriate for those with limited life expectancy or at risk of iatrogenic hypoglycaemia

GLYCOSYLATED HAEMOGLOBIN (OR FRUCTOSAMINE)

Glycosylated haemoglobin, or HbA1c, is formed by the non-enzymatic glycation of part of the β-chain of haemoglobin. HbA1c levels correlate to the *mean* plasma glucose over the preceding 9–10 weeks. The relationship between HbA1c and mean plasma glucose levels is shown in Table 3.2. A recent HbA1c result should normally be available at the full periodic review. HbA1c should be checked more frequently when control is poor or glycaemic management has been altered. The estimation of HbA1c requires expensive equipment and stringent quality control: it is generally not feasible in primary care and is best done by a hospital laboratory.

Serum fructosamine levels, if available, correlate to the *mean* plasma glucose over the preceding 1–2 weeks and may serve as an alternative if the HbA1c is not "valid", such as in the presence of anaemia or a haemoglobulinopathy.

PATIENT SELF-MONITORING

Achieving and maintaining good glycaemic control usually requires effective patient self-monitoring and/or monitoring by his carer. Health education is an essential component of self-monitoring. The patient needs to be motivated and able to test accurately, interpret the results correctly and act upon them appropriately: this can only be achieved by regular patient education. Self-monitoring results should be recorded and brought to any diabetes review where glycaemic control is discussed.

Urine testing

Testing urine for the presence of glucose using test strips, such as Diabur-Test 5000, is non-invasive, inexpensive and may be preferred by patients who dislike blood testing,

TABLE 3.2 Correlation between HbA1c level and mean plasma glucose levels (Rohlfing et al 2002)

HbA1c (%)	Mean plasma glucose level (mmol/l)
6	7.5
7	9.5
8	11.5
9	13.5
10	15.5
11	17.5
12	19.5

although there is some recent evidence that patients with type 2 diabetes can have negative perceptions about urine testing (Lawton 2004).

However, urine glucose testing has two main drawbacks:

1. The quantity of glucose, if any, in a sample of recently formed urine is more indicative of the mean blood glucose levels over the period of time when the urine was formed than of the blood glucose level at a given moment. Urine levels of glucose do not reflect any sudden fluctuation in blood glucose levels and are, thus, inexact.
2. In some type 2 patients, the renal threshold for glycosuria is abnormally high or low. Thus, it is possible for no glycosuria to be present with a moderately raised blood glucose level, or for glycosuria to be present with a normal blood glucose level.

Despite these limitations, if adequate glycaemic control (i.e. good HbA1c, infrequent hypoglycaemia) is achieved with urine testing, then blood testing may be unnecessary in type 2 diabetics on diet alone or oral medication. Once diabetic control is stable, the urine should usually be negative for glucose. If it becomes persistently raised (e.g. more than 2% on four consecutive days) or the patient becomes ill, professional advice should be sought.

Blood testing

Blood glucose testing is recommended for diabetics treated with insulin (both types 1 and 2), but may be desirable in patients on diet alone or oral medication, who require accurate blood glucose estimations. Blood glucose testing is more expensive than urine testing, and requires the correct use of a properly calibrated blood glucose meter and appropriate education to develop self-confidence in interpreting and acting upon test results.

Many varieties of finger-pricking lancets, blood glucose machines and test strips or sensors are now available, but only the lancets and strips/sensors can be prescribed on the NHS. Each different make of blood glucose machine has its own unique test strips. The current issue of the Monthly Index of Medical Specialities (MIMS) lists each make of test strip and the machine(s) with which it is compatible. There have been significant technical advances in machines, with sensors allowing the blood drop to be analysed outside the machine. A rigorous evaluation of the different blood glucose meters and lancing devices now available on the UK market was published in 2005 by the Department of Health's Medicines and Healthcare products Regulatory Agency (details can be downloaded from its website, *www.mhra.gov.uk*). This useful source should assist in selecting the most suitable machine or device. Recently the MHRA has identified a safety problem with some blood glucose meters, where units of measurement may change and mislead the user.

Although blood glucose machines are not currently available on prescription, many are inexpensive, often costing less than £20 (the manufacturers' main profit is in the sale of the test strips or sensors). If the GP writes a letter simply confirming the diagnosis of diabetes in a named patient, then that patient is exempt from paying Value Added Tax (VAT) when purchasing his machine, provided that the machine is intended for that patient's personal use. Lancets need to be disposed of safely; preferably using either a needle clip or a sharps bin (both can be prescribed).

There is a consensus that patients on insulin should undertake daily self-monitoring of blood glucose to adjust insulin doses and avoid hypoglycaemia. Depending on the insulin regimen and other factors, the recommended frequency may be up to four or five times daily. For those on oral medication or diet only, there is variable evidence that blood glucose self-monitoring improves glycaemic control. If the risk of hypoglycaemia is small, measuring HbA1c levels may be the best way to monitor glycaemic control. When the HbA1c is less than 7.5%, routine self-monitoring of blood glucose offers little benefit. If control is not stable, then self-monitoring of blood glucose may be helpful, provided that it is "supported by appropriate education and advice" (Drug and Therapeutics Bulletin 2007).

Plasma glucose values are 11% higher than whole blood glucose values. Machines will be calibrated to either of these. The blood glucose targets for good control are 4–7 mmol/l pre-meal and < 10 mmol/l post-meal. If glycosuria or raised blood glucose is found, an increased dose of either the oral blood glucose-lowering drug or insulin may be appropriate. Dietary energy intake, if excessive, should be reduced. If the medication is given in divided doses, the dose that covers the tested time of day must be adjusted accordingly. However, if after stabilisation and despite adjustment of treatment, the blood glucose becomes > 20 mmol/l for more than 4 days, or if the patient becomes ill, then he should seek medical help urgently. Persistently abnormal levels should prompt a review of the balance between medication, diet and physical activity.

PATIENT SYMPTOMS

Patient well-being is a much less precise and a potentially misleading method of assessing glycaemic control, particularly as **hyperglycaemia** is not always symptomatic. However, most professionals and patients recognise that abolition or reduction of diabetic symptoms, such as polydipsia, diuresis, blurred vision and fatigue is both necessary and desirable.

Recurrent **hypoglycaemia** indicates poor glycaemic control; these episodes may occur when there has been an error in dosage of blood glucose-lowering medication (usually insulin), a small or missed meal or unplanned exercise (when medication dosage has not been correctly reduced). Sometimes, there is no apparent cause for hypoglycaemia.

BLOOD GLUCOSE-LOWERING MEDICATION

In patients with type 2 diabetes, there is likely to be a progressive deterioration over time of pancreatic β-cell function, resulting in most patients eventually requiring insulin to achieve acceptable glycaemic control. The main classes of oral blood glucose-lowering medication act by improving either insulin secretion (insulin secretagogues) or insulin action. For a drug to stimulate insulin secretion, it is necessary for the pancreatic β-cells to still be functioning. Further details about the drug classes discussed below can be found in the *British National Formulary* (BNF, section 6.1.2).

A stepped approach to achieving and maintaining metabolic control is sensible. Starting with lifestyle changes and the early introduction of monotherapy, it moves progressively onto logical and effective combinations of different agents if the HbA1c remains greater than 7.0%. This is summarised in Table 3.3, with more than one option at some numbered steps, choice depending upon the clinical circumstances and patient preference (ADA 2007). It is the authors' personal view that, in primary care, basal insulin is best introduced only when maximal oral therapy (including triple therapy, if feasible) cannot achieve good metabolic control.

Changes to treatment should be guided not only by a recent HbA1c, but also self-monitoring results, opportunities to optimise lifestyle and the patient's well-being and concordance. The interval between any dose changes must allow sufficient time for their effect to be seen, but prompt action is indicated in the event of repeated hypoglycaemia or significant hyperglycaemia. Ideally, additional medication should be introduced only after the maximum recommended dose of current medication has failed to achieve reasonable glycaemic control or is not tolerated.

Other medical problems must be managed appropriately. If uncertain about any aspect of management, it is sensible to seek specialist help.

INSULIN SECRETAGOGUES (DRUGS THAT IMPROVE INSULIN SECRETION)

Currently, there are two main groups of drugs that increase insulin secretion:

1. *Sulphonylureas*, some of which have been available for many years

   and

2. *Post-prandial regulators of glucose (PPRGs)*, also known as *meglitinide analogues*. These have been introduced more recently and have a rapid onset and short duration of action.

NICE's *Clinical Guidelines* in 2002 recommended that "a generic sulphonylurea should normally be the insulin secretagogue of choice" (NICE 2002).

Sulphonylureas

This class of drugs acts by stimulating insulin secretion from pancreatic β-cells (although there is less stimulation of first-phase secretion than by the PPRGs), but do not affect insulin resistance. In the absence of ketonuria, sulphonylureas are indicated in nonobese patients whose blood glucose is not controlled by diet. Sulphonylureas can be combined with either metformin, a glitazone, basal insulin or acarbose. The following agents are available: *tolbutamide, glibenclamide (glyburide), gliclazide* (also available in a modified-release formulation), *glimepiride, gliquidone, glipizide* and *chlorpropamide*. Sulphonylureas should be introduced slowly with the dose titrated according to self-monitoring and HbA1c results.

The different sulphonylureas appear to have a comparable effect upon blood glucose-lowering, but with different durations of action. Although both once-daily and twice-daily dosing are associated with better concordance, once-daily preparations

TABLE 3.3 Summary of the stepped treatment of raised blood glucose in type 2 diabetes

At each numbered step, letter "a" is first choice option, subject to drug contraindications, clinical circumstances and patient preference.

Step	Evaluation	Intervention
1	HbA1c <7.0%	Lifestyle advice (diet and physical activity)
2a	a. HbA1c ≥7.0% b. Absence of significant renal (eGFR <45 ml/min), hepatic or cardiac impairment or risk of sudden deterioration	Metformin
2b	a. HbA1c ≥7.0% b. Metformin not tolerated or contraindicated	Insulin secretagogue (usually sulphonylurea) or glitazone (alternative in renal impairment)
3a	HbA1c ≥7.0% on first-line drug (maximum tolerated dose)	Combination of: metformin and insulin secretagogue (usually sulphonylurea)
3b	a. HbA1c ≥7.0% on first-line drug (maximum tolerated dose) b. Insulin secretagogue not tolerated or likely high level of insulin resistance	Combination of: metformin and glitazone
4a	a. HbA1c ≥7.0% (but less than 8.0%) on two oral drugs (maximum tolerated doses) b. Very obese or unwilling to consider insulin therapy c. Absence of contraindications	Combination of metformin and sulphonylurea and rosiglitazone
4b	a. HbA1c ≥7.0% on two oral drugs (maximum tolerated doses) b. Triple therapy not tolerated/ contraindicated or unlikely to work (very raised HbA1c)	Add basal insulin*
5	HbA1c ≥7.0% on combination of basal insulin and oral agent(s)	Intensify insulin regimen (consider adding rapid- or short-acting)

*Of the two glitazones, only pioglitazone currently has a licence to be prescribed in combination with insulin.

have the advantages of reducing the total number of tablets that a patient needs to take and of potentially simplifying the drug regimen.

Sulphonylureas are contraindicated in severe hepatic and renal impairment, porphyria, during breast feeding and pregnancy, or when ketoacidosis is present. The short-acting tolbutamide can be used in renal impairment, as can gliclazide and gliquidone, which are metabolised mainly in the liver.

The two main drawbacks associated with sulphonylureas are that they can induce hypoglycaemia and can encourage weight gain. Glibenclamide is associated with the rare but potentially fatal occurrence of nocturnal hypoglycaemia in the elderly. Weight gain was recorded with both chlorpropamide and glibenclamide (but less than with insulin) in the intensively treated group of patients in the UKPDS (UKPDS 1998). However, hypoglycaemia and weight gain are not inevitable with sulphonylureas, and the risks of either occurring may be minimised by:

- Avoiding the long-acting agents, chlorpropamide (no longer recommended) and glibenclamide.
- Avoiding use in patients with mild to moderate hepatic and renal impairment, and being careful about use in the elderly (shorter-acting agents are safer and to be preferred).
- Careful introduction and dose titration of the drug (according to the results of self-monitoring and HbA1c).
- Using the lowest dose that achieves and maintains normoglycaemia.

The side-effects of sulphonylureas are mild and infrequent, and include gastro-intestinal disturbances and hypersensitivity reactions (a skin rash that usually appears within 6–8 weeks of initiation).

Post-prandial regulators of glucose (PPRGs)

These drugs are also known as *meglitinide analogues* or *rapid-acting insulin secretagogues*. The two available drugs in this group are *repaglinide* and *nateglinide*. Both can be used in combination with metformin, but nateglinide is not currently licensed for monotherapy.

The main action of PPRGs is to increase (more than sulphonylureas) the first-phase insulin secretion in response to rising plasma glucose levels by pancreatic β-cells, with the effect of reducing the mealtime "glucose spike". PPRGs are best initiated at an earlier stage in the disease process, when pancreatic β-cells have more capacity to secrete insulin. PPRGs have a quicker onset (usually within 15 minutes) and shorter duration of action (up to 3 hours) than sulphonylureas. Nateglinide appears to have a slighter quicker onset and shorter duration of action than repaglinide. PPRGs may be preferable to sulphonylureas in a patient who either wishes or needs to fast (e.g. during Ramadan), or whose meal times are unpredictable and/or irregular.

PPRGs should be avoided in patients with severe liver disease or on dialysis, and in pregnancy, breast feeding and ketoacidosis. Their side-effects include hypoglycaemia, particularly in elderly patients and in those with adrenal or pituitary insufficiency (probably less risk than with sulphonylureas) and hypersensitivity reactions. Weight gain is also possible, although less so than with sulphonylureas. Other side-effects reported with repaglinide include gastro-intestinal disturbances, rash and visual disturbances. Nateglinide interacts with ACE inhibitors, diuretics and corticosteroids.

DRUGS THAT IMPROVE INSULIN ACTION

Biguanides

Metformin is the only available drug in this class. It remains the first-choice drug in obese type 2 diabetics and a first-line option in the non-obese. Metformin acts by decreasing gluconeogenesis in the liver and by increasing glucose uptake in peripheral tissues. Its excretion is entirely renal and it has a short half life. Metformin is not associated with either weight gain or serious hypoglycaemia. Metformin can be combined with all secretagogues, both glitazones and the different insulins.

In addition to its efficacy in helping to achieve and maintain glycaemic control, metformin has been shown to increase survival, particularly in the obese. In the UKPDS study, treatment with metformin was shown to reduce all-cause mortality by 36%, compared to treatment with either insulin or a sulphonylurea (UKPDS1998). This is why metformin remains the first-line oral hypoglycaemic agent.

Metformin's main side-effects are on the gastrointestinal tract; these can be minimised by a stepped approach to increasing the dose and by the medication being taken with or after food. Strict adherence to all the published contraindications, related to a perceived increased risk of precipitating lactic acidosis is not supported by systemic reviews (Salpeter et al 2002), and would result in metformin being prescribed only rarely, despite its undoubted value to many patients.

There is a slight risk of precipitating lactic acidosis with metformin in vulnerable individuals. Specific contraindications and guidelines for withdrawing metformin now include (Jones et al 2003, modified by authors):

- If impaired renal function develops: reduce dose (maximum 500 mg twice daily) if serum creatinine is >130 μmol/l; stop if serum creatinine is >200 μmol/l.
- Avoid if hepatic (such as those with alcohol dependence) or cardiac (if there is concurrent treatment with a β-blocker) "impairment" are present.
- Withdraw during periods of suspected tissue hypoxia (e.g. through myocardial infarction, sepsis or respiratory failure).
- Withdraw for 3 days after contrast medium that contains iodine has been given and reinstate when renal function is normal and stable.
- Withdraw 2 days before general anaesthesia and reinstate when renal function is normal and stable.

As this guidance was published before the Renal NSF, clinicians may need to revisit the definition given above for renal impairment. It is reasonable to reduce metformin dose if the eGFR is <60 ml/min and to stop metformin if the eGFR is <45 ml/min, but any decision must balance the benefits against the risks. Metformin is contraindicated in people with heart failure; however, it has been suggested recently that metformin may not only be safe, but may potentially improve clinical outcomes (Eurich et al 2005). Further studies are required to clarify this issue.

As a precaution, some experts recommend regular renal monitoring (serum creatinine or eGFR) and serum B12 estimations in patients on long-term metformin.

Glitazones or thiazolidinediones (TZDs)

These are also known as peroxisome proliferator-activated receptor-gamma (PPAR-γ) agonists (Krentz et al 2000). They act by promoting glucose utilisation peripherally, which enhances insulin action, but does not affect insulin secretion. Glitazones are thought to activate nuclear receptors, located mainly in adipose tissue, that affect glucose and lipid metabolism, and to maintain insulin secretion by pancreatic β-cells (Day 1999) by reducing the effect of glucose "toxicity". Once initiated, it may take 6–10 weeks for glitazones to work fully.

The two currently available glitazones, *rosiglitazone* and *pioglitazone*, were launched in the UK in 2000. *Troglitazone* was launched in the UK in October 1997 and voluntarily withdrawn by its manufacturers weeks later, following reports of serious hepatic reactions worldwide. Current evidence suggests that neither rosiglitazone nor pioglitazone are hepatotoxic, but liver function should be monitored. These drugs are licensed as monotherapy, in combination with either metformin OR a sulphonylurea, or in triple therapy with metformin AND a sulphonylurea (only rosiglitazone is licensed for triple therapy). Their current UK licence does not include prescribing in combination with meglitinide analogues, but pioglitazone can now be prescribed in combination insulin. When compared with placebo, both glitazones significantly reduced HbA1c levels, either as monotherapy or in combination with other anti-diabetic agents (Chiquette et al 2004). Glitazones can cause weight gain, in part through fluid retention, which may precipitate heart failure, particularly if a glitazone is combined with insulin. Recently there have been reports of a rare association between glitazones and the development of macular oedema.

The use of glitazones has been the subject of debate and evolving guidance since their launch; possibly in part because both agents are very expensive when compared to metformin or to most sulphonylureas. Additionally, recent publications have raised concerns about the adverse affects of glitazones on cardiovascular outcomes, as well as the increased risk of fractures in women (Richter 2007). The NICE Appraisal Committee issued guidance first in 2000/1, then updated in August 2003 on the use of both rosiglitazone and pioglitazone within their current UK licences. NICE recommends their use mainly in those unable to take metformin and a sulphonylurea in combination because of lack of tolerance or a contraindication to one of these drugs (NICE Appraisal Committee 2003). However, in September 2003 the European Agency for the Evaluation of Medicinal products (EMEA) extended the licence of glitazones as preferred second-line drugs in addition to metformin in obese patients (Bailey et al 2003).

In 2004, the Association of British Clinical Diabetologists (ABCD) produced a position statement that included the following recommendations for patients with type 2 diabetes (Higgs et al 2004):

- A glitazone is the preferred second-line oral agent in addition to metformin in the obese.
- A glitazone can replace metformin in renal impairment.
- A glitazone is not a substitute for insulin if poor control on maximal tolerated metformin and sulphonylurea combination.
- Triple therapy, with rosiglitazone, metformin and a sulphonylurea, may be considered in the very obese or in patients unwilling to go onto insulin.

- Glitazones should not be used in combination with insulin, in heart failure, or in patients with pre-treatment serum transaminase levels more than 2.5 times the upper limit of normal.

In obese type 2 patients (particularly from some ethnic groups), insulin resistance is likely to be significant. This needs to be tackled by a combination of nonpharmacological (improving diet and levels of physical activity) and pharmacological interventions. If monotherapy with metformin fails to achieve adequate glycaemic control, then, as the next step, a metformin–glitazone combination may be preferred to a metformin–sulphonylurea combination, since sulphonylureas do not reduce insulin resistance.

Possibly the greatest benefit comes from using glitazones earlier in the natural history of type 2 diabetes when there is more pancreatic β-cell activity. The NICE guidelines warn that the substitution of a glitazone for a first-line drug, after failure of the metformin–sulphonylurea combination, does risk an initial worsening of glycaemic control, which may not be recoverable. Introducing insulin at this stage may be preferable to the substitution with a glitazone.

In assessing the effect of glitazones on cardiovascular risk factors, a meta-analysis found that pioglitazone had a better effect than rosiglitazone on lipids (rosiglitazone increased LDL-C and total cholesterol and had no effect on TG levels; pioglitazone had no effect on LDL-C or total cholesterol and lowered TG levels), although both significantly increased HDL-C. No significant differences were shown between rosiglitazone and placebo in changes to systolic or diastolic blood pressure. Both glitazones are associated with weight gain (Chiquette et al 2004).

Looking at "hard" cardiovascular outcomes:

- The PROactive Study recruited 5238 type 2 diabetics with existing CVD (excluding heart failure), comparing treatment with 45 mg pioglitazone against placebo (plus existing glucose-lowering and other medications in both groups). It reported that over 3 years in the treatment group there was a statistically significant absolute risk reduction of 2.1% (NNT = 48) for a pre-specified secondary composite event rate consisting of all-cause mortality, nonfatal myocardial infarction (excluding silent myocardial infection), and stroke. However, there was no statistically significant difference between the two groups in the primary (mixed medical and surgical) endpoint for which the study was powered (Dormandy et al 2005). The interpretation of the clinical outcomes' data is still under debate (Freemantle 2005).

There are two studies involving rosiglitazone:

- The ADOPT study recruited 4360 drug-naïve subjects, comparing treatment with rosiglitazone or metformin or glibenclamide on disease progression, β-cell function, risk markers for macrovascular complications over 4 years. The primary outcome was time to monotherapy failure (defined as a confirmed fasting plasma glucose >10 mmol/l. The cumulative monotherapy failure was 15% for rosiglitazone, 21% for metformin and 34% for glibenclamide. Rosiglitazone was associated with more weight gain and oedema than either metformin or glibenclamide, but with fewer gastro-intestinal side effects than metformin and less hyperglycaemia than glibenclamide (Kahn 2006).

- The RECORD study, due to report in 2009, recruited 3966 subjects, inadequately controlled on either metformin or sulphonylurea, comparing treatment with rosiglitazone plus metformin or sulphonylurea against metformin plus sulphonylurea on cardiovascular outcomes. An interim analysis in June 2007 was inconclusive (although under-powered) about differences in the risk of MI or CVD death, but found an increased risk for heart failure in the rosiglitazone-treated group (Home 2007).

Two recently published meta-analyses show a significantly increased risk for MI in type 2 diabetics treated with rosiglitazone (Nissen 2007; Psaty 2007), not found in individual trials. This needs clarification, but it is unlikely that rosiglitazone reduces CVD risk. The latest MHRA advice is not to discontinue rosiglitazone abruptly, but to review its use at the next routine appointment (MHRA 2007). In light of the above and the recent launch of new agents (see page 81), the future use of glitazones is likely to decline. Patients benefit most from optimizing <u>both</u> glycaemic control and cardiovascular risk factors: neither should be managed at the expense of or while ignoring the other.

OTHER ORAL DRUG THERAPY

Alpha-glucosidase inhibitors

The only drug in this class currently available in the UK is *acarbose* (Glucobay). It inhibits intestinal alpha-glucosidase, delaying the digestion of starch and sucrose which increase blood glucose levels after carbohydrate ingestion. The result is a fall in post-prandial glucose and insulin levels. Acarbose can be prescribed either as monotherapy or in combination with other oral agents. It does not cause weight gain and is unlikely to cause hypoglycaemia as monotherapy. Its widespread use is limited by gastrointestinal side-effects, which occur in up to 60% of patients. These are dose dependent, and include flatulence, bloating and diarrhoea. As these occur most frequently at the initiation of treatment, careful titration may reduce their incidence. Acarbose is best taken with meals rich in starch. It should be considered as an alternative in patients unable to use the other oral drugs. Acarbose is expensive.

INSULIN

Clinical indications for changing to insulin in type 2 diabetes

Pancreatic β-cell secretion declines as the type 2 diabetes progress; therefore, most type 2 diabetics will eventually need to be transferred onto insulin. Clear prior explanation should prevent patients who arrive at this point from feeling either guilty or a "failure".

The indications for changing to insulin include:

- Intolerance of and/or inadequate response to oral hypoglycaemic agents
- Contraindications to oral therapy
- Acute symptoms of hyperglycaemia or intercurrent illness and/or steroid therapy, which can exacerbate hyperglycaemia
- Continual weight loss (in the presence or absence of ketones)
- Poor healing and/or recurrent infection

- Post myocardial infarction
- Pregnancy.

Insulin preparations

A wide variety of insulin preparations is currently available. Insulins can be classified according to their onset and duration of action, summarised in Table 3.4. They also vary according to their origin and method of manufacture (animal-derived,

TABLE 3.4 Overview of insulin preparations (revised from Krentz 2001)

Category	Generic types	Proprietary examples	Onset of action (minutes)	Peak of action	Duration of action (hours)
Rapid-acting	Lispro, aspart, glulisine	Humalog, NovoRapid, Apidra	15 15 10–20	40–60 minutes	3–5
Short-acting	Regular*	Actrapid, Velosulin Hypurin, Humulin S, Insuman Rapid	15–60	1–3 hours	4–8
Rapid-acting and intermediate-acting	Biphasic insulin aspart, Biphasic insulin lispro	NovoMix30, HumalogMix 25 or 50	10–20	2 peaks (as for its components)	12–18
Short-acting combined with intermediate-acting (biphasic)	Regular – isophane (NPH) mixture	Mixtard 10–50, Humulin M3, Hypurin 30, InsumanComb 15, 25, 50	15–60	2 peaks (as for its components)	12–18
Intermediate-acting (basal)	Isophane (NPH)	Insulatard, Hypurin, Humulin I, Insuman Basal	60–120	4–8	12–18
Long-acting	Crystalline zinc suspensions (insulin zinc suspension)	Monotard, Hypurin Lente, Ultratard	120–240	6–18	18–>24
Newer prolonged-acting	Insulin glargine, insulin detemir	Lantus, Levenmir	150	Plateau	23

*The term "soluble" no longer applies to short-acting insulins only, since prolonged preparations (such as insulin glargine) have become available

semisynthetic or synthetic), modifications that alter the duration of action, and their mode of delivery (e.g. syringe, pen, infusion device).

Onset and duration of action

Different pharmaceutical companies have adopted different names for the same insulins or their mixtures. Further details are available in the latest issues of both the BNF (Section 6.1.1) and MIMS (Section 7A).

1. Rapid-acting insulins:

    These recently developed insulin analogues (amino acid substitutions) have both a more rapid onset and shorter duration of action than the traditional "short-acting" insulins. Further details are in the subsection below on modifications to insulin. Two preparations are available currently, lispro and aspart. Their onset is quick (within 5–10 minutes), their peak of action is early (within 1 hour) and their duration of action is brief (3–5 hours). The optimal time to inject is just as a meal begins. These insulins are particularly used in a basal bolus regimen.

2. Short-acting insulins:

    Ideally, short-acting insulin should be given 30–45 minutes before meals to match its peak action to glucose absorption from the gastrointestinal tract. A delayed meal risks hypoglycaemia and injecting just before, during or after a meal will not facilitate tight glycaemic control, as the insulin's onset of action may occur after it is most needed. In these circumstances, rapid-acting insulin may be more suitable and effective.

3. Intermediate-acting insulins:

    The *isophane* preparations, also known as neutral protamine Hagedorn (NPH), are produced by complexing insulin with protamine. Although they can be used as monotherapy either once or twice daily, they are often mixed with either rapid- or short-acting insulins. They can also be given as a single bedtime dose, combined with daytime oral agents in patients with type 2 diabetes (see below). For convenience, premixed insulins (also known as biphasic) are available, containing both short- or rapid-acting and intermediate-acting insulins (e.g. Mixtard, Humulin M and Humalog Mix) in various proportions. In European nomenclature the short-acting percentage is given in the preparation's proprietary name. The 30% mixture is often favoured in the UK.

4. The long-acting insulins:

    These are becoming less popular, because their mixture with short-acting insulins causes problems, and because premixed and prolonged-acting analogue insulins have now become available and are being increasingly preferred.

Origin and method of manufacture

Short-, intermediate- and long-acting insulins are either based on the human sequence of amino acids or extracted from an animal pancreas, usually porcine (less antigenic than beef), and then purified. Synthetic human insulin is produced either by enzyme modification of porcine insulin (emp) or, more commonly, from a proinsulin synthesised by bacteria (prb) or from a precursor synthesised by yeast (pyr). Human insulins have a more rapid onset and shorter duration of activity than porcine insulins (Krentz 2001).

Modifications that alter the onset and duration of action

Genetically engineered insulin analogues that contain modifications to soluble human insulin have been introduced. These include:

1. **Rapid-acting**, have a rapid onset and a short duration of action. There are three available in the UK:
   - *lispro* transposes two amino acids, lysine and proline, on the B chain to B28 lysine and B29 proline
   - *aspart* (aspartate replaces proline at B28)
   - insulin *glulisine* appears to have a slightly quicker onset of action than lispro and aspart.
2. **Prolonged-acting**. There are currently two basal insulin analogues available in the UK. Both have a prolonged plateau of concentration rather than a peak (less risk of hypoglycaemia); and both have a duration of activity just under 24 hours, a once-daily injection can often cover a patient's daily basal insulin needs. Because of these features, the new analogues may potentially replace isophane as the basal insulin of choice:
   - Insulin *glargine* (two additional arginine molecules are placed at B31 and B32, at the C terminus of the B chain, and arginine replaces asparagine at A21, making the molecule more stable). Insulin glargine should be administered in the evening or at bedtime. When converting to insulin glargine from isophane, the dosage should be 20% less than the total 24 hour dose of the previous basal insulin. Insulin glargine was the subject of a NICE Technology Appraisal in 2002 (NICE 2002).
   - Insulin *detemir* (Levemir) was launched in the UK in 2004. It is administered once or twice daily. When converting from isophane to insulin detemir, the total dosage does not require adjustment if the pre-meal blood glucose averages 6.5 mmol/l or less; however, the total dosage should be increased by 10%, 20% and 25% if the pre-meal blood glucose averages, respectively, 6.6–10 mmol/l, 10.1–15 mmol/l and > 15 mmol/l. When both pre-breakfast and pre-dinner targets cannot be reached, then consider splitting the total daily insulin detemir dose into two injections.

Both basal insulin analogues can be used either on their own or in combination with oral agents (metformin or sulphonylurea), or with short- or rapid-acting insulin.

Possible insulin regimens

The insulin regimen used has to be tailored to the patient's needs and lifestyle, and it must take into account the patient's wishes and sensitivities. Rapid-, short-, intermediate- and long-acting insulin preparations may be injected either separately or mixed together in the same syringe.

Three regimens are commonly used:

1. *Combination of a basal* (intermediate-acting or prolonged-acting) *insulin* once or twice daily *AND oral hypoglycaemic drug*(s) during the day. This may be no more effective than insulin alone, but the combination may be more practical for some

patients. Omitting the oral agent and administering once daily basal insulin may be appropriate for those patients (e.g. a frail, isolated elderly diabetic) in whom tight blood glucose control is not the main therapeutic goal or where hypoglycaemia may be disastrous. Insulin glargine or insulin detemir may provide a flatter plateau than isophane.

2. *Twice-daily insulin* before meals in the morning and evening. This regimen is usually a combination of intermediate-acting insulin (often two-thirds of the total daily dose is given before breakfast and one-third before the evening meal or at bedtime) AND a rapid- or short-acting insulin, either drawn up separately or as a pre-mixed combination. Insulin can be combined with metformin. Sometimes better glycaemic control can be achieved using different preparations for the morning and evening injections. The usual starting dose is 8 to 10 units twice daily, with titration until glycaemic targets are reached. However, this titration can be accelerated by using slide rules, devised by the UKPDS. These calculate the total insulin dose likely to be required by any diabetic, based upon gender, fasting blood glucose, height and weight. The initial total insulin dose should be one-half to two-thirds of the calculated likely final total insulin dose. A drawback of an accelerated increase of insulin dose is greater weight gain when compared to the conventional slower insulin dose titration.

3. The *basal bolus regimen* is increasingly popular because of its flexibility. Rapid-acting insulin is administered before each main meal, with either twice-daily intermediate-acting or a single injection at bedtime of prolonged-acting insulin (e.g. insulin glargine or detemir). If using a pre-mixed combination of rapid- and intermediate-acting insulin twice daily, it is still possible to give an additional dose of rapid-acting insulin in-between to cover a large meal.

There is good evidence that better glycaemic control, weight loss and reduced risk of hypoglycaemia are more likely when combining metformin and insulin.

Insulin dose adjustment

Insulin doses need to be titrated against blood glucose levels, aiming for 4–7 mmol/l before meals. It may take a few weeks to achieve normal blood glucose levels. Due to insulin resistance, some type 2 diabetics may eventually require very large doses of insulin (greater than 2 units/kg body weight/day) to achieve and maintain adequate glycaemic control.

Principles of dose adjustment

Although the circumstances and needs of each patient on insulin may vary, a few guiding principles should help:

- Try to avoid changing insulin on the basis of a one-off reading
- Review also monitoring and injection techniques, eating and activity levels and patterns
- Consider time distribution, as well as quantity and type of insulin to be administered
- Look for patterns: identify periods of the day with greatest problems
- Agree finite dose changes, e.g. 2 units, and allow an interval of a few days between dose changes to allow the patient time to adapt and ascertain effect.

Practical guidance for different regimens

For a twice-daily regimen using a free-mixing regime:

- If glucose is high or low *before breakfast*, increase or decrease *evening long-acting* insulin
- If glucose is high or low *before lunch*, increase or decrease *morning short-acting* insulin
- If glucose is high or low *before supper*, increase or decrease *morning long-acting* insulin
- If glucose is high or low *before bed*, increase or decrease *evening short-acting* insulin.

For a twice-daily regimen using a fixed biphasic insulin regime:

- If glucose is high or low *before breakfast*, increase or decrease *evening* insulin dose
- If glucose is high or low *before supper*, increase or decrease *morning* insulin dose
- Other adjustments probably require a change in the mixture's components.

For a basal bolus regimen:

- If glucose is high or low *before breakfast*, increase or decrease *evening long-acting* insulin
- If glucose is high or low *before lunch*, increase or decrease *morning rapid-acting* insulin
- If glucose is high or low *before supper*, increase or decrease *lunchtime rapid-acting* insulin
- If glucose is high or low *before bed*, increase or decrease *teatime rapid-acting* insulin.

Over insulinisation

Recurrent hypoglycaemia, weight gain, wildly variable blood glucose values and subtle features of chronic hypoglycaemia (headache, personality change in elderly, the need to eat) suggest a chronic overdose of insulin.

How to make the change to insulin

It may be best to seek expert advice before initiating insulin. Unless the patient is ill, insulin can be started on an outpatient basis. The professional responsible should have the appropriate knowledge and skills, allocate sufficient time to address all of the patient's needs and agenda, and remain accessible to monitor progress and provide support.

If the primary care team takes charge, an agreed and effective protocol should be followed. Success is possible: in one of the authors' practice, the average HbA1c of the first 15 patients transferred onto insulin dropped from 9.7 to 6.9% (Curley, personal communication). Some innovatory teams have looked at a group approach, in which six to 10 patients can attend together, with the benefits of increased cost-effectiveness and of greater mutual support between often-anxious individuals in a similar situation.

In assessing the person who requires insulin, the following issues should be considered:

- *Implications to lifestyle*. Patients who switch to insulin are no longer eligible for a group 2 driving licence and for certain jobs.
- *Level of support at home*. This is particularly important if dexterity and/or vision are impaired and the patient may not be able to administer his or her own insulin.
- *Cultural and religious beliefs*. For example, animal-derived insulins are unacceptable to Muslims, Jews and strict vegans. The insulin regimen used must avoid hypoglycaemia when the patient is required to fast.
- *Psychological and physical health issues*. In very obese insulin-resistant patients, insulin may cause further weight gain. Many type 2 diabetics who switch to insulin may be frightened of needles and may regard the switch as a "failure". A clear explanation of the likely benefits that arise from good diabetic control with a demonstration using a syringe or pen may go some way to alleviating these fears.

Key educational points for insulin conversion

Clear and correct advice on the following aspects of self-administering insulin should be given to patients, and suitable written literature should be made available for reference (Avery & Moore 1999).

Equipment: choosing a suitable injection device

The choice is between a disposable U100 insulin syringe with an attached needle and one of the wide range of pen-injector devices. Both have their respective advantages and disadvantages. Staying in touch with a friendly diabetes specialist nurse should enable the primary care team to keep up-to-date with developments. MIMS is a useful source of information about the syringes, pen needles and most pens that are available free on FP10 prescription. Syringes are smaller and lighter than pens, but pens are more portable, may be more suitable for those with visual problems and the patient does not need to carry a vial of insulin to be drawn up for each injection. Both syringes and pens require some degree of manual dexterity to use.

Mixing insulins

If free-mixing insulins, the short-acting preparation must be drawn into the syringe *before* the intermediate-acting preparation to avoid contamination of the short-acting vial with protamine or zinc.

Injection technique

The injection technique is as important as the type of insulin injected or the device used. The three key factors that influence insulin absorption are depth, site and technique (see Table 3.5):

Subcutaneous *depth* is preferred for everyday use, but the distribution of subcutaneous tissue can vary between ages, sex, body mass distribution and site. Appropriate needle size is important to avoid the injection being either too shallow (intradermal) or too deep (intramuscular or another structure).

TABLE 3.5 Guidance for choosing appropriate needle size and injection technique (Wilbourne 2002) © John Wiley & Sons Ltd; reproduced with permission

Patient	Injection technique	Needle size (mm)
Overweight adult	Pinch-up, 90°	12.7
	No pinch-up, 45°	12.7
	No pinch-up	8
Normal-weight adult	Pinch-up, 90°	8
Thin adult	No pinch-up, 90°	5 or 6
Children, adolescents	No pinch-up, 90°	5 or 6

Sites should be rotated and, for reliable absorption, different areas should not be used simultaneously. Injections should be spaced out within each area, moving one finger-breadth from the previous site:

- thighs (anterior or lateral) have a slow absorption speed and are suitable for intermediate-acting insulin
- the abdomen (the whole of the anterior abdominal wall) has a fast absorption speed and is suitable if fast-acting absorption is required
- arms (upper external quadrant) have a medium-to-fast absorption and require shorter needles
- buttocks (upper outer quadrants) have slow absorption.

Technique:

- The skin needs to be pinched (between flexed thumb and index or middle finger) when the injection is given at 90°
- Choose the right needle size
- Avoid insulin leakage by waiting 5–10 seconds after the injection to withdraw the needle, doing so as pinch-up is released
- Inject usually 20–30 minutes before eating, but rapid-acting insulin should be injected just before a meal
- Good hygiene of site, hands and equipment is essential.

Other points:

- Clear instructions about diet are essential and suitable carbohydrate intake between meals may be necessary to prevent hypoglycaemia.
- Care of equipment, storage, keeping spares, noting expiry dates and *correct disposal of sharps* (using a safe-clipper or sharps container – both prescribable) *and syringes* (can also use sharps container) according to local council guidelines (e.g. in screw-top plastic bottles).

- Drivers must inform the Driver and Vehicle Licensing Agency (DVLA) and driving insurance company of the change.
- Patients should be taught to recognise the causes and features of hypoglycaemia. They should be advised to carry both treatment (glucose sweets or fruit drink followed by longer-acting carbohydrates) and identification (card, necklace or bracelet) at all times.

Inhaled insulin

The first inhaled insulin, *Exubera*, gained FDA approval in January 2006 and was launched in the UK in May 2006. This was a short-acting or prandial insulin that was administered via the lungs by oral inhalation using an insulin inhaler. Its action profile was similar to the rapid-acting insulins. Although patients still needed to administer their usual subcutaneous basal insulin (either intermediate or long-acting), not surprisingly, patient satisfaction for the use of inhaled insulin appeared to be greater than for injected insulin, regardless of whether inhaled insulin was added to oral agents or subcutaneous insulin therapy (Capelleri 2002). The main drawbacks of inhaled insulin were:

- its contra-indications (hypoglycaemia, poorly controlled or severe asthma, severe COPD, current or recent (duration of cessation less than 6 months) smoking and pregnancy) and'
- its cost.

In December 2006 NICE published its guidance that "inhaled insulin is not recommended as a routine treatment for people with type 1 or type 2 diabetes" and should be a specialist (NICE 2006). On 18 October 2007, Exubera's manufacturer (Pfizer) announced that it would no longer be making Exubera "available to patients". Pfizer stated that it based its decision on commercial reasons and not on any safety problems.

No other inhaled insulin is currently available in the UK.

POSSIBLE FUTURE DEVELOPMENTS IN BLOOD GLUCOSE-LOWERING TREATMENT

Fixed-dose combinations

Fixed-dose combinations of established oral blood glucose-lowering agents may return to favour and become available in the UK, if only to improve compliance by reducing the number of tablets patients have to swallow. Both glitazones are now available in combination with metformin: avandment (rosiglitazone) and competact (pioglitazone). Other combinations that may come onto the UK market include:

- *Gliovance* – metformin and glibenclamide (glyburide in the US), available in the US
- *Metaglip* – metformin and glipizide.
- *Avandaryl* – rosiglitazone and glimepride

Improving insulin release

A number of new approaches with the potential to enhance insulin secretion are being explored or are about to become available. These include:

Incretin mimetics

The fact that oral glucose leads to greater insulin secretion than a comparable intravenous glucose load suggests that the gut may produce hormone(s) that increase this secretion. The intestinal hormone *glucagon-like peptide-1* (GLP-1) has a number of actions:

1. Binding to pancreatic islet β-cells to stimulate insulin secretion, dependent on the presence of elevated blood glucose
2. Inhibition of glucagon secretion, also dependent on the presence of elevated blood glucose
3. Delaying gastric emptying and reducing gastric motility
4. Reducing appetite (a central effect of unknown mechanism)
5. Acting directly on β-cell growth and survival.

GLP-1 has an extremely brief plasma half-life and duration of action, and is degraded rapidly by the proteolytic enzyme dipeptidyl peptidase IV (DPP-IV).

Two pharmaco-therapeutic approaches to exploit the actions of GLP-1 have been used:

1. GLP-1 analogues that are resistant to DPP-IV. These are administered by subcutaneous injection.

    Exenatide, the first available mimetic agent, is administered twice daily. At its launch, Exenatide has been licensed in combination with metformin and/or a sulphonylurea, but not with a glitazone or insulin, or as monotherapy. It is excreted renally and should not be administered if eGFR is less than 30. The main side effects are nausea, vomiting, diarrhoea, feeling jittery, headache, dizziness and dyspepsia. Exenatide was approved in the US in 2005 and launched in Europe in 2007. A long-acting formulation of exenatide, Exenatide LAR, is currently undergoing clinical trials. Another agent, Liraglutide, is derived from modifying GLP-1 by coupling it with a fatty acid. Several other compounds are in different stages of development. Since these drugs are "glucose-dependent", they act only when blood glucose is raised, reducing the risk of hypoglycaemia.
2. Selective inhibition of DPP-IV enzymes (which have other substrates apart from GLP-1 and other actions, including suppression of glucagon release).

    These oral agents are called "gliptins". In 2007 *Sitagliptin* became available in the UK. A second agent, *Vitagliptin*, is likely to follow in 2008. *Sitagliptin* is a once daily agent and is currently licensed to be taken in combination with either metformin or a glitazone, but not with a sulphonylurea or as monotherapy. Both drugs improve glycaemic control. A third agent, Saxagliptin, has recently entered phase 3 clinical trials. Various other compounds are in different stages of development. The long-term safety (due to their complex and various actions) and precise clinical role are still not entirely clear.

Other potential therapeutic approaches

- *Succinate esters* targeted at beta cells to stimulate proinsulin biosynthesis and insulin secretion by enhancing the Krebs cycle
- *Imidazoline compounds*
- *Phosphodiesterase inhibitors* targeted at β-cells, which might promote insulin secretion by other agents.

Alternative insulin delivery systems

In view of many diabetics' distaste for and fear of injections, scientists have been seeking alternative ways for patients to receive insulin. Two promising areas are:

- Different routes of insulin administration (e.g. via nasal mucous membranes or via inhalation – see above for details about *Exubera*). A new technology is AERx, which is an "electronic pulmonary delivery system" that Novo Nordisk are developing to administer insulin by inhalation
  and
- Transplantation of donor islet cells that would then produce insulin in response to blood glucose levels, but preventing rejection requires expensive medication that has its own side effects.

METABOLIC EMERGENCIES

HYPOGLYCAEMIA

NSF
7

Definition

Hypoglycaemia is an abnormally low blood glucose level that leads to symptoms of sympathetic nervous system stimulation or of central nervous system dysfunction.

Causes

The causes of hypoglycaemia in patients with type 2 diabetes are:

- Drug induced, such as by insulin, sulphonylureas, repaglinide, alcohol
- Missed or small meal
- Unplanned exercise
- Combination of the above.

Interventions

The interventions include:

- *Prevention* by education of the patient and close family members on the warning symptoms; timing of medication, meals and physical activity; the need to always carry identification and/or a warning card or bracelet and "instant carbohydrate".
- *Confirm* by testing blood glucose, ideally using an accurate blood glucose machine.

- *Immediate correction* of low blood glucose – if conscious and co-operative, use "instant carbohydrate"; otherwise inject glucagon (ensure the family has a device and the instructions).
- If a patient suffers from repeated hypoglycaemia, an *evaluation* of diet, lifestyle and drug treatment, followed by appropriate adjustments, is necessary.

HYPEROSMOLAR NONKETOTIC HYPERGLYCAEMIC COMA

The syndrome *hyperosmolar nonketotic hyperglycaemic coma* (HONK) is a complication of type 2 diabetes and is characterised by hyperglycaemia, extreme dehydration and hyperosmolar plasma (without significant ketonuria or acidosis).

The onset is often insidious with nonspecific symptoms such as confusion and drowsiness, and including features of dehydration (particularly if hyperglycaemia is accompanied by inadequate fluid intake). HONK presents usually in patients aged over 60 years and up to 40% of cases occur without a previous diagnosis of diabetes. There is usually a precipitating medical condition, such as myocardial infarction or sepsis. HONK has a very high mortality rate, particularly in frail and/or socially isolated patients.

The diagnosis is based upon marked hyperglycaemia (usually greater than 50 mmol/l) and a calculated osmolality (2 [Na + K] + glucose) greater than 350 mosmoles. Serum bicarbonate is usually greater than 15 mmol/l and urinary ketones should be ++ or less on dip-stick testing. Treatment is immediate hospital admission to correct fluid balance and biochemistry. These patients are often very insulin-sensitive, but may require insulin for a few weeks. During admission they usually need anticoagulation, due to the high risk of thromboembolic disease.

▶ KEY POINTS

- The combination of self-monitoring results, a recent HbA1c result, and the patient's well-being should guide glycaemic treatment.
- Due to the progressive deterioration of pancreatic cell function, a step-up approach may be useful in prescribing medication. Most type 2 diabetics will eventually require insulin to achieve acceptable glycaemic control.
- Metformin, sulphonylureas and glitazones are the main oral glycaemic drug classes used.
- Insulin is now available in a wide variety of types, formulations and delivery systems: these can be tailored to a regimen suitable for each individual.
- Conversion to insulin in primary care can be successful if proper training (of both patient and professional) occurs and a suitable insulin regimen is chosen. Education is essential to enable the patient to self-manage insulin optimally.
- There are a number of promising new developments in drug treatment.
- Hypoglycaemia and hyperosmolar nonketotic hyperglycaemic coma are significant metabolic complications and require prompt effective treatment.

REDUCING CARDIOVASCULAR RISK

OVERVIEW

Since the origin of much diabetes-related morbidity and mortality is vascular, reducing cardiovascular risk is an important aim in the management of type 2 diabetes. Following a preliminary discussion of cardiovascular risk, each of the main treatable cardiovascular risk factors (rationale, assessment, targets and interventions) is reviewed.

There is strong evidence to support the efficacy of modifying cardiovascular risk factors to prevent or delay the onset and development of cardiovascular disease (CVD). Whilst careful attention needs to be paid to the assessment and modification of individual risk factors, for any "high-risk" individual (which includes all people with type 2 diabetes), the greatest benefit will come from attacking aggressively all relevant risk factors, irrespective of the baseline, and not from an excessive focus on one factor to the possible exclusion of others: in other words, a broadly based approach. This approach is followed in the most recent guidelines from the Joint British Societies (Wood et al 2005) and the American Diabetes Association (ADA 2007). Readers may also find it useful to refer to a 2006 review by Marshall and Flyvbjerg published in the *BMJ* (Marshall & Flyvbjerg 2006).

The section ends with a brief survey of the important non-treatable risk factors and an "alternative" view of targets.

UNDERSTANDING CARDIOVASCULAR RISK

The incidence of atheromatous disease is much greater in the diabetic than general population. It is the devastating effects of this atheromatous disease that require effective and aggressive interventions, aimed at minimising future mortality and morbidity. There is considerable evidence to support an approach that assumes, for type 2 diabetics, that prevention needs to be **secondary** (CVD is present) rather than **primary** (CVD is absent), even in those without any manifestation or evidence of vascular disease. To prevent future CVD, asymptomatic patients may have to undergo potentially unpleasant or even dangerous treatment. Such interventions are more likely to be appropriate and justifiable if both the concept of risk and the factors contributing to increased risk are understood.

DEFINITIONS

Risk can be defined as the probability or expected frequency of harmful effects (due to a biological agent) occurring over a defined period of time.

Although risk can be expressed in different ways, it is useful to understand the difference between absolute and relative risk:

- The *absolute risk* of a particular event occurring over a specified period of time is usually expressed either as a percentage (*a* %) or a ratio (*b* incidences per a defined population size).

- *Relative risk* is usually expressed as a particular event being *c* % or *d* times more or less likely to occur in a defined population than in a compared population over a specified period of time.

Where the absolute risks of two compared events or interventions are very low, small differences of risk may be relatively "large". For example, if a treatment reduces the risk of an adverse event occurring from 2% to 1%, then the absolute risk reduction is an unimpressive 1%, but the relative risk reduction is a staggering 50%: this fact does not escape copywriters in advertising.

The results of a risk–benefit analysis of an intervention are often presented now as "number needed to treat" (NNT). NNT is the reciprocal of absolute risk reduction. If a treatment reduces absolute risk by 1 in 10 or 10%, then the NNT of that treatment is 10. NNT is a better, much less misleading, representation of a treatment's effectiveness than relative risk reduction.

Although the term *vascular* can refer to the whole of the circulatory system, it is sometimes used to refer to a part of the system. In order to be precise, the term vascular should be qualified in such circumstances to indicate which part of the circulation is being described. When considering the long-term vascular complications of diabetes, it is useful to subdivide these according to vessel size into:

- *Macrovascular* – coronary heart disease, cerebrovascular disease and peripheral arterial disease

  and

- *Microvascular* – retinopathy, nephropathy and neuropathy.

Discussions about vascular risk relate mostly to macrovascular disease, and the distinction needs to be made between:

- *Coronary heart disease (CHD) risk,* which refers to the probability of developing CHD

  and

- *CVD risk,* which refers to the probability of developing all forms of macrovascular or cardiovascular disease: a combination of the risks for developing coronary heart disease, cerebrovascular disease and peripheral arterial disease.

These concepts are relevant when quantifying and describing risk.

WHAT FACTORS ARE ASSOCIATED WITH CARDIOVASCULAR RISK IN PATIENTS WITH DIABETES?

Different parameters, characteristics or factors contribute, both individually and collectively, to the overall cardiovascular risk in any single individual, particularly one with diabetes. Not all factors affect cardiovascular risk equally, nor are all of them independent or susceptible to modification.

Cardiovascular risk factors can be divided into nonmodifiable and modifiable (see Table 4.1). Only modifiable factors can respond to intervention. However, some nonmodifiable risk factors are needed to calculate global cardiovascular risk and, if present, can serve as a prompt to help identify those individuals in whom this risk should be assessed and "tackled", particularly in people normally considered to be at lower risk, such as those *without* diabetes.

Of the modifiable risk factors for CVD, smoking, raised blood pressure and dylipidaemia are generally regarded as the most important, both for their contribution to overall cardiovascular risk and for the resultant reduction of that risk when "corrected".

Although individual risk factors may have an independent effect upon the global cardiovascular risk, their overall effect upon cardiovascular risk is often more than additive, with different risk factors combining "at times … to become permissive for harm or create harm greater than that effected by simple addition" (Simmons 2002). In 1993 the MRFIT study demonstrated that the greater than additive adverse effect of a collection of risk factors is especially marked in diabetes, where the increase in risk attributed to any single or combination of risk factors is doubled when compared to a nondiabetic population (Stamler et al 1993). There are still gaps in the evidence base. Matters become more complicated when evaluating the efficacy of various interventions.

It is important to move away from focussing on a single risk factor to the exclusion of others. There are recognised situations or scenarios where risk factors are clustered, e.g. metabolic syndrome. Interventions that concentrate upon modifying a single risk factor may be much less effective in reducing cardiovascular risk than in adopting a multi-factorial approach.

TABLE 4.1 Cardiovascular risk factors and markers in people with diabetes mellitus

Non-modifiable risk factors	Modifiable risk factors
Age	Smoking status
Gender	Raised blood pressure
Ethnic group	Dyslipidaemia
Family history	Lack of physical activity
	Poor diet
	Obesity
	Poor glycaemic control
	Excess alcohol
	Elevated fibrinogen
	Cardiomyopathy
	Raised inflammatory markers
	Microalbuminuria
	Hyperhomocysteinaemia

TABLE 4.3 Target blood pressure levels for diabetics recommended by different organisations

Blood pressure target (mmHg)	Learned body/organisation	Date published
145/85	New GP Contract	2003, reviewed 2006
140/90	NICE (North of England 2004)	August 2004
140/90	NICE (NICE 2006a)	June 2006
140/80	SIGN (SIGN 2001)	November 2001
140/80	National Clinical Guidelines for Type 2 Diabetes (Hutchinson et al 2002)	October 2002
140/80	UKPDS 36 (Adler et al 2000)	2000
130/80 (optimal)	British Hypertension Society Guidelines	2004
140/80 (acceptable)	BHS-IV (Williams 2004)	
130/80	American Diabetes Association (ADA 2007)	January 2006
130/80	JBS 2 (Wood et al 2005)	December 2005

A variety of automated sphygmomanometers are now available. Before purchasing any model, the buyer is advised to enquire whether the device has passed independent validation using the protocols of the British Hypertension Society (BHS) and the Association for the Advancement of Medical Instrumentation Standard (AAMI) (O'Brien et al 2001). Additional useful advice may be available from the local hospital's medical physics department. Further independent evaluation of the available blood pressure measuring devices is being undertaken and may be published at some point in the future.

The use of mercury sphygmomanometers is *still* legal (the problems arise with safe disposal of mercury). When set up properly they can be as accurate as the best automated machine. Many aneroid sphygmomanometers lose accuracy when jolted.

Due to pressures of time and less than ideal ergonomics, many health professionals do not invariably measure a patient's blood pressure correctly. Detailed authoritative guidance on how it should be done is given in Table 4.4, a counsel of perfection. To minimise inaccuracies, some key points to remember when measuring blood pressure include:

1. Use the correct-sized cuff.
2. Ensure the arm is supported, the patient is quiet and his legs are not crossed.
3. Arrhythmias render any blood pressure measurement less reliable.
4. Daytime ambulatory blood pressure values average 10/5 mmHg less than surgery measurements.

TABLE 4.4 Guidelines for Blood Pressure Measurement (from North of England 2004, O'Brien et al 2003, British Hypertension Society website)

Blood pressure measurement: procedure

Measure sitting blood pressure routinely: standing blood pressure should be recorded at least once at the initial estimation

Try to standardise the procedure:
   remove tight clothing
   relaxed temperate setting, with the patient seated (ideally for at least 5 minutes prior to measurement)
   position arm for measurement out-stretched, in line with mid-sternum, and supported at heart level
   avoid talking during measurement
   use a properly maintained, calibrated, and validated device

Correctly wrap a cuff containing an appropriately sized bladder around the upper arm and connect to a manometer. Cuffs should be marked to indicate the range of permissible arm circumferences; these marks should be easily seen when the cuff is being applied to an arm

Palpate the brachial pulse in the antecubital fossa of that arm

Rapidly inflate the cuff to 20 mmHg above the point where the brachial pulse disappears

Deflate the cuff and note the pressure at which the pulse re-appears: the approximate systolic pressure

Re-inflate the cuff to 20 mmHg above the point at which the brachial pulse disappears

Using one hand, place the stethoscope over the brachial artery ensuring complete skin contact with no clothing in between

Slowly deflate the cuff at 2–3 mmHg per second listening for Korotkoff sounds. Read blood pressure to the nearest 2 mmHg:
   Phase I: The first appearance of faint repetitive clear tapping sounds gradually increasing in intensity and lasting for at least two consecutive beats: note the **systolic pressure**
   Phase II: A brief period may follow when the sounds soften or "swish"
   Auscultatory gap: In some patients, the sounds may disappear altogether
   Phase III: The return of sharper sounds becoming crisper for a short time
   Phase IV: The distinct, abrupt muffling of sounds, becoming soft and blowing in quality
   Phase V: The point at which all sounds disappear completely: note the **diastolic pressure**

When the sounds have disappeared, quickly deflate the cuff completely

When possible, take readings at the beginning and end of consultations. Take the mean of at least two readings. More recordings are needed if marked differences between initial measurements are found

5. Readings can vary significantly between arms, time of day and different days.
6. Beware of the "white coat effect" (readings can be raised when taken by health-care professionals) (MHRA 2006).

Target organ damage

Any evidence of target organ damage should be sought. The "organs" to consider are the eyes (retinopathy), kidneys (proteinuria, renal impairment), heart (left ventricular hypertrophy) and feet (neuropathy, impaired circulation and/or foot ulcer).

Potential causes of hypertension

If there are any underlying causes of hypertension, is the lifestyle (diet, alcohol, smoking, lack of exercise) a contributory factor? Some types of medication can cause raised blood pressure, such as cold cures, hormone replacement therapy, oral corticosteroids, nonsteroidal anti-inflammatory drugs, and carbenoxolone. Examination occasionally reveals palpable kidneys (which could indicate polycystic kidneys or an adrenal mass), renal bruits (which may indicate renovascular disease) and delayed or absent femoral pulses (which occur in co-arctation of the aorta).

Family history

The family history should be checked for hypertension, vascular or renal disease, particularly in first-degree relatives (parents, siblings or children).

Investigations

In addition to routine diabetic investigations (eGFR, lipid profile, urinary albumin: creatinine ratio), requesting an ECG, an echocardiogram (if available) or a renal ultrasound may provide useful information. However, referral to a specialist may be indicated for further investigations to inform management, particularly when there are concerns or when treatment targets are not achieved.

INTERVENTIONS: OVERVIEW

The main aims here are to reduce the overall cardiovascular risk and prevent diabetes complications.

When is treatment indicated?

A single measurement is rarely sufficient to ascertain an individual's "true" blood pressure level and, thus, to justify a decision on whether to treat. Repeated measurements need to be taken over a length of time (the 2006 NICE guidelines recommend at least two further separate readings). The duration of observation prior to a treatment decision depends upon how elevated the measurements are, and if target organ damage and/or any other vascular risk factors are present. If the measurements are elevated only slightly and there is no target organ damage in a "low-risk" individual, it is reasonable to observe over several months. If the measurements are elevated markedly or target organ damage is present in a "higher-risk" individual, a briefer duration of observation with earlier intervention is indicated.

If there is considerable variation between measurements or if there is the possibility of "white coat" hypertension, it may prove helpful to undertake 24-hour ambulatory blood-pressure monitoring, if available.

INTERVENTIONS: NONPHARMACOLOGICAL METHODS

Nonpharmacological methods of reducing blood pressure are worth undertaking. As for all diabetic patients, those with raised blood pressure should be urged to not smoke, restrict alcohol, reduce salt intake, take more exercise and eat healthily, aiming for weight loss if obese. Good glycaemic control reduces vascular risk.

INTERVENTIONS: PHARMACOLOGICAL METHODS

The huge range and quantity of blood-pressure-lowering drugs available mirrors that of blood glucose-lowering medication. Before discussing the individual drug classes, several key concepts need to be borne in mind:

- Apart from likely efficacy, a number of factors may influence which drug is chosen as first-line.
- In many patients, more than one drug will be required to gain and maintain adequate blood pressure control.
- The actual level of blood pressure achieved is as important as which class of drug is used.
- Blood pressure control should be achieved within the context of correcting all relevant modifiable cardiovascular risk factors.

In support of the Diabetes NSF, the National Clinical Guidelines for type 2 diabetes published its recommendations for the pharmacological management of raised blood pressure in 2002 (Hutchinson et al 2002). However, these have been superseded by the 2006 guidelines from NICE (NICE 2006a), and the 2005 JBS 2 guidance on the prevention of CVD. The Quality and Outcomes Framework of the GMS contract sets a unified threshold for intervention and target (see Appendix 3).

Blood pressure reviews

Blood pressure should be checked not only at the full periodic diabetes review, but also at the interim review (every 4–6 months). If there is an intervention, the interval between blood pressure reviews should be shorter, every 1–3 months, and any side effects monitored.

Referral

Referral is indicated if:

- An underlying cause of hypertension or if an abnormality on physical examination is found

- Blood pressure achieved with a suitable combination of drugs is still significantly above target
- Target organ damage (particularly kidneys) is present.

Drug classes for the treatment of raised blood pressure

Five classes of blood-pressure-lowering drugs have been shown to be effective in reducing cardiovascular mortality and morbidity in patients with type 2 diabetes and raised blood pressure:

1. Angiotensin converting enzyme (ACE) inhibitors
2. Angiotensin II receptor blockers (ARB)
3. Beta (β) blockers
4. Nondihydropyridine and long-acting dihydropyridine calcium channel blockers (CCB)
5. Thiazide and thiazide-like diuretics (Clinical Evidence online, ADA 2004).

Although some of the supporting evidence came from trials comparing treatments against placebo, more data are now available comparing different effective treatments or combinations. An overview of this evidence is found in Table 4.5. The trials cited below are referred to by their acronyms, with their full names given in Appendix 5. The indications, cautions and contraindications for the major classes of antihypertensive drugs are summarised in Table 4.6.

In addition, there are other drug classes of blood-pressure-lowering drugs that are sometimes used in patients with diabetes:

- alpha-1 adrenergic blockers
- potassium-retaining diuretics (spironolactone)
- other antihypertensive agents (the rest).

Further details of the names and dosages of different blood-pressure-lowering agents are given in Appendix 1 and in the BNF Section 2.

Angiotensin converting enzyme (ACE) inhibitors

This drug class blocks the conversion of angiotensin-I to angiotensin-II (a powerful vasoconstrictor and an indirect facilitator of the sympathetic nervous system) by inhibiting the angiotensin converting enzyme. This produces a reduction in angiotensin-II levels, leading to arteriolar and venous dilatation and a fall in blood pressure. The antihypertensive effect of ACE inhibitors is dose-related.

Angiotensin-II has other actions that are thought to be harmful to the cardiovascular system, contributing to the pathogenesis of large and small vessel structural changes in hypertension and other CVD (Luft 2001). ACE inhibitors also suppress aldosterone secretion, increase renal blood flow (producing natriuresis) and increase circulating levels of bradykinin, a vasodilating cytokine which can cause cough. ACE inhibitors have little effect upon heart rate or airways resistance. ACE inhibitors have no adverse effects upon lipid metabolism or glucose tolerance, but there have been reports that they may be less effective in Afro-Caribbean patients. Drugs in this class have generic

TABLE 4.5 Summary of studies of antihypertensive therapies in type 2 diabetes

Study	Description	Outcome	Diabetes sample size
ABCD	Enalapril vs. nisoldipine	Greater MI event + mortality with nisoldipine	470
ALLHAT	Chlorthalidone vs lisinopril, and amlodipine	Thiazides prevented more CVD (1 or more forms)	15 297
ASCOT	Amlodipine +/– perindopril +/– vs. atenolol +/– bendroflumethiazide	Amlodipine +/– perindopril more effective in reducing stroke, all cardiovascular events, and cardiovascular mortality	2532
CAPP	Captopril vs. β-blocker or diuretic	Captopril group had fewer MI + lower mortality	572
CHARM	Candesartan vs. placebo	Candesartan significantly reduced cardiovascular deaths and hospital admissions for heart failure	57
FACET	Fosinopril vs. amlodipine	Both treatments reduced BP, but fewer events on fosinopril	380
HDFP	Stepped care vs. referred care	More active treatment reduced total CVD + mortality	772
HOPE	Ramipril vs. placebo	Ramipril prevented events + mortality	3577
HOT	Felodipine + other agents to target diastolic BP < 90, < 85, < 80 mmHg	Lower BP produced greatest reduction in CVD events	1501
INVEST	Verapamil (sustained release) vs. atenolol (trandolapril and/or hydrochlorothiazide added to achieve target)	No statistically significant difference between groups in either BP control or CVD events	6400
LIFE	Losartan vs. atenolol	Losartan prevented more CVD mortality + events	1195
NORDIL	Diltiazem vs. β-blocker or diuretic	Similar efficacy	727
SHEP	Chlortalidone vs. placebo	Chortalidone prevented more events and reduced total mortality	583
STOP-2	ACE vs. CCB vs. conventional treatment	Similar efficacy	719

TABLE 4.5 Summary of studies of antihypertensive therapies in type 2 diabetes

Study	Description	Outcome	Diabetes sample size
SYST-EUR	Nitrendipine vs. placebo	Treatment reduced CVD + mortality	492
SYST-CHINA	Nitrendipine vs. placebo	Treatment reduced CVD	98
UKPDS	Captopril vs. atenolol	Similar efficacy	758

TABLE 4.6 Compelling and possible indications, contraindications and cautions for the major classes of antihypertensive drugs (Wood et al 2005)

Class of drug	Compelling indications	Possible indications	Cautions	Compelling contraindications
ACE	Heart failure, LV dysfunction, post-MI, CHD, type 1 diabetic nephropathy, secondary CVA prevention	Chronic kidney disease, type 2 diabetic nephropathy, proteinuric renal disease	Renal impairment, PVD	Pregnancy, renovascular disease
ARB	ACE intolerance, type 2 diabetic nephropathy, hypertension with LVH, heart failure in ACE-intolerant people, post-MI	LV dysfunction post-MI, intolerance of other antihypertensive drugs, proteinuric renal disease, chronic renal disease, heart failure	Renal impairment, PVD	Pregnancy, renovascular disease
Beta-blockers	MI, angina	Heart failure	Heart failure, PVD, diabetes (except with CHD)	Asthma, COPD, heart block
DCCB	Elderly, ISH, angina, CHD	Elderly, angina, MI		
CCB (rate-limiting)			Combination with β-blockade	Heart failure, heart block
Thiazide / thiazide-like diuretics	Elderly, ISH, heart failure, secondary stroke prevention			Gout
Alpha-blockers	Benign prostatic hypertrophy		Postural hypotension, heart failure	Urinary incontinence

names ending in "-pril". They include *captopril, cilazapril, enalapril, fosinopril, imidapril, lisinopril, moexipril, perindopril, quinapril, quinopril, ramipril* and *trandolapril*.

Class side-effects include:

- Persistent cough in 10 to 20% of users (greater in East Asians)
- Angio-oedema in about 1% (threefold greater in Afro-Caribbeans)
- Taste disturbance
- Rash.

ACE inhibitors should not be prescribed to women who are likely to become pregnant, due to the teratogenic risk of foetal renal maldevelopment, nor to patients with bilateral renal artery disease, as this might precipitate deterioration in renal function leading to renal failure. Concurrent prescribing of ACE inhibitors with potassium supplements or potassium-sparing diuretics should be avoided, unless specifically required and with careful electrolyte monitoring.

Initiating an ACE inhibitor can produce a sharp fall in blood pressure in patients when the renin-angiotensin system is activated (e.g. when dehydration, heart failure, or accelerated hypertension are present), but this sudden drop is rarely seen in uncomplicated hypertension. Although renal artery stenosis may be detected by the presence of a renal artery bruit, it is often sub-clinical. As a precaution, serum eGFR or creatinine should be checked within 2 weeks of initiating an ACE inhibitor in order to detect any loss of renal function early enough to stop the drug and prevent significant irreversible deterioration. A change of less than 10% from the baseline value is not clinically significant.

The ABCD (Estacio et al 1998) and FACET (Tatti et al 1998) studies found ACE inhibitors to be superior to dihydropyridine calcium channel blockers in preventing cardiovascular events in type 2 diabetics. ACE inhibitors have been shown to improve cardiovascular outcomes in high cardiovascular risk patients with diabetes, independently of whether hypertension was present (HOPE 2000, PROGRESS 2001). In the ASCOT study, the treatment group, in which the ACE inhibitor perindopril was the add-in drug, achieved lower blood pressures, had fewer CVAs and total CVD events, and lower all-cause mortality (Dahlöf et al 2005). Some of these differences could be attributed to the lower blood pressure levels achieved and improvements in other cardiovascular risk factors in this group. ASCOT was stopped early due to differences in mortality between the two treatment groups: as a result, it lacked sufficient power to detect a statistically significant difference between the groups for the primary endpoint (nonfatal MI or CHD death).

Angiotensin II receptor blockers (ARB)

This drug class blocks type I angiotensin-II (AT1) receptors. These drugs are less likely than ACE inhibitors to cause cough or angio-oedema, due to their selectivity for the AT1 receptor and their lack of potentiation of bradykinin and possibly other vasopeptides. Therefore, ARBs may be suitable for patients in whom ACE inhibitors are not tolerated.

Drugs in this class have generic names ending in "-sartan". Currently available are *candesartan, eprosartan, irbesartan, losartan, olmesartan, telmisartan* and *valsartan.* Cautions and contraindications are the same as for ACE inhibitors. Both ACE inhibitors and ARB conserve renal function in diabetic nephropathy and are beneficial in heart failure.

In the LIFE study, an ARB was superior to a β-blocker in improving CVD outcomes in a subset of patients with diabetes, hypertension and left ventricular hypertrophy (Dählof et al 2002, Lindholm et al 2002). In the CHARM study, candesartan improved cardiovascular outcomes against placebo (Pfeffer et al 2003). The candesartan and lisinopril microalbuminuria (CALM) study (Mogensen et al 2000) suggested that the combination of the ACE inhibitor lisinopril with the ARB candesartan may be more effective in reducing blood pressure and urinary albumin excretion than the individual drugs in type 2 diabetics (although the study dose of lisinopril was only half the maximal dose).

Beta (β) blockers

The antihypertensive effect of beta-blockers is not completely understood. β1-blockers competitively inhibit β-adrenoreceptors in the heart. β2-blockers inhibit β-adrenoreceptors in peripheral vasculature, bronchi, and elsewhere. β-blockers decrease heart rate (negative chronotropic effect), the force of cardiac muscle contraction and cardiac output (negative inotropic effect), and renin secretion. Some β-blockers may have direct CNS activity, although this is not necessarily responsible for their blood-pressure-lowering effect. In addition to their established role in treating hypertension and angina, some β-blockers are now used to treat heart failure. They are also used to relieve some symptoms of anxiety, in the prophylaxis of migraine, and topically in glaucoma.

The different β-blockers now available (generic names end in "-lol") vary in:

1. *Duration of action*: shorter-acting β-blockers may need to be given two to three times daily. Modified-release formulations may be suitable as once daily in treating hypertension. Some β-blockers (e.g. *atenolol, bisoprolol, carvedilol, celiprolol,* and *nadolol*) have a longer duration of action, allowing a once-daily regimen.
2. *Selectivity for β1-receptors* (cardioselectivity): the first-generation β-blockers (e.g. *propranolol* and *oxprenolol*) are noncardioselective. The second-generation β-blockers (e.g. *atenolol, bisoprolol* and *metoprolol*) tend to be more cardioselective.
3. *Lipid or water solubility*: some are lipid soluble and some are water soluble. *Atenolol, celiprolol, nadolol,* and *sotalol* are the most water-soluble; they are less likely to enter the brain and cause CNS disturbances (e.g. lethargy, impaired concentration and memory, vivid dreams). Since water-soluble β-blockers are excreted renally, dosage reduction may be necessary in renal impairment to prevent accumulation.
4. *Partial agonist activity* (also known as intrinsic sympathomimetic activity or ISA): β-blockers with ISA (e.g. *acebutolol, oxprenolol* and *pindolol*), similarly to the more

cardioselective β-blockers, are less likely to cause peripheral vasoconstriction and have lesser negative chronotropic and ionotropic effects.

5. *Effects on metabolism*: first-generation β-blockers can exacerbate metabolic abnormalities (increased triglyceride and reduced HDL-C levels, and reduced hepatic glucose mobility, especially when combined with thiazide diuretics). The second-generation β-blockers have a less (but still demonstrable) adverse effect upon serum triglyceride and HDL-cholesterol levels. The third-generation β-blockers (e.g. *celiprolol* and *nebivolol*) are not thought to have an adverse effect upon plasma lipids.

These differences may influence choice in treating particular diseases or individual patients, although they are *not* invariably or equally relevant clinically.

The third-generation β-blockers (e.g. *celiprolol* and *nebivolol*) have a peripheral vasodilating effect. The cardiac remodelling effects of sympathetic nervous system dysfunction in the heart may be prevented or minimised by the use of β-blockers, especially third-generation agents such as carvedilol. This action may be responsible for the reduction in morbidity and mortality in patients with diabetes reported in heart failure trials. Combined receptor antagonists (e.g. *carvedilol* and *labetalol*) act on both α- and β-receptors. The α-blocking activity offsets peripheral vasoconstriction and the adverse effect on plasma lipids produced by β-blockade.

All β-blockers should be avoided in patients with obstructive airways disease (asthma or bronchospasm) and used with caution in diabetes treated by insulin (risk of masking the symptoms of imminent hypoglycaemia). β-blockers can also cause erectile dysfunction.

Recently, doubts have been cast on whether the β-blocker atenolol does reduce cardiovascular mortality and stroke in hypertensive patients, despite its proven blood-pressure-lowering effect (Carlberg et al 2004). Because atenolol has been used as a reference drug in many studies, it is unclear whether these reservations apply to atenolol alone or to other β-blockers as well. β-blockers are not recommended as first-line drugs for "routine treatment" in the 2006 NICE guidelines.

However, the following need to be borne in mind:

- The actual reduction of blood pressure per se is important.
- Drug combinations including β-blockers are frequently required to achieve target blood pressure levels.
- β-blockers are important in treating angina and heart failure, frequently present in diabetics.
- β-blockers are safe and recommended in women who are fertile and could become pregnant.
- β-blockers have important benefits in secondary prevention post-myocardial infarction.

Other currently available β-blockers not mentioned above are *esmolol, nadolol*, and *timolol*.

Calcium channel blockers (CCB)

This drug class blocks voltage-dependent calcium channels on the surface of cell membranes, preventing the influx of calcium ions into the cell and reducing the availability of intracellular calcium for muscle contraction; leading to reduced vascular tone and decreased peripheral vascular resistance; and a fall in blood pressure. The most important of the six known types of calcium channel in the cardiovascular system is the long-lasting (L-type) channel, found in all excitable cells, including the vasculature, myocardium and cardiac conducting tissue.

L-type CCBs can be subdivided into three different classes:

- **Class I**, phenylalkylamines (e.g. verapamil). They depress cardiac conduction and may precipitate heart failure if there is AV or SA node dysfunction or if prescribed concurrently with β-blockers. Verapamil has an additional anti-arrhythmic action.
- **Class II**, dihydropyridines, abbreviated as DCCB (e.g. amlodipine, felodipine, isradipine, lacidipine, lercanidipine, nicardipine, nifedipine and nisoldipine). They are relatively selective for the blocking L-type channels in smooth muscle cells, thus inducing vascular relaxation with a fall in vascular resistance and arterial pressure. They do not depress conduction or contractility; thus, they are much less likely to precipitate heart failure. They may be used safely in combination with β-blockers. The main side effects of DCCBs are vasodilator: dose-dependent peripheral oedema (resulting from transudation of fluid from vascular compartments into the dependent tissues due to pre-capillary arteriolar dilatation), headache, flushing, palpitations and gum hypertrophy. These side effects can sometimes be offset by dose titration or by the use of slow-release or long-acting drugs such as amlodipine, lacidipine or lercanidipine.
- **Class III**, benzothiazepines (e.g. diltiazem). This class has a slightly negative or negligible ionotropic effect.

Both class I and III CCBs are sometimes referred to as nondihydropyridine CCBs. All three CCB classes do not affect plasma lipids or glucose metabolism, and are effective in elderly and black patients.

Bioavailability is an important factor to consider when prescribing sustained-release preparations of CCBs. Different preparations containing the same quantity of a given drug are unlikely to have identical pharmacokinetic profiles. It is recommended that such preparations are prescribed by their proprietary name and that patients are not transferred to another preparation without assessment and titration.

A prospective randomised, blinded trial suggested that ACE inhibitors were more effective than CCBs at preventing myocardial infarction in hypertensive patients with diabetes and concerns were raised over the safety of CCBs (Estacio et al 1998). At the European Society of Cardiology meeting in 2000, Furberg and his colleagues presented their meta-analysis of several trials, finding no difference in the blood pressure levels achieved by CCBs and other drug classes, but suggested that patients receiving CCBs were at increased risk from certain major cardiovascular events (a question of safety or of efficacy?). The National Clinical Guidelines for Type 2 Diabetes in 2002, recommended prescribing long-acting (avoid short-acting) CCBs only as second-line treatment or as part of combination therapy (Hutchinson et al 2002). The INVEST study found that patients with CHD and hypertension (even in the diabetic subgroup) had a similar reduction in CVD mortality if treated with either verapamil or atenolol (Pepine et al 2003). ASCOT reported DCCBs to be safe and effective (Dahlöf et al 2005). The British Hypertension Society did not express concerns about the safety or efficacy of CCBs in their 1999 (Ramsay et al 1999) and 2004 (Williams 2004): DCCBs are one of the three drug class options recommended as first line by NICE in its 2006 guidelines.

Thiazide/thiazide-like diuretics

These lower blood pressure by complex mechanisms. Their antihypertensive effect is thought to be mediated by arteriolar vasodilatation. This is partly due to the urinary loss of sodium that results from a blockade of renal tubular reabsorption of sodium. Reflex vasoconstrictor activation (including the renin-angiotensin-aldosterone system) may accompany the early loss in blood volume induced by thiazides, resulting in a temporary increase in peripheral resistance. However, following initiation of a thiazide, further blood pressure lowering will occur over a period of days as peripheral resistance gradually decreases. The antihypertensive dose-response to thiazides is flat and they should be prescribed at the lowest effective dose. The duration of diuresis differs from the duration of antihypertensive effect.

Thiazide diuretics include *bendroflumethiazide, chlorthiazide, cyclopenthiazide, hydrochlorothiazide, hydroflumethiazide* and *polythiazide* (generic drug names end in "-thiazide"). They may differ from thiazide-like diuretics (these include *chlortalidone* and *indapamide*) in their duration of action, ion calcium-blocking activity, and carbonic anhydrase inhibitory activity. The significance of these differences is uncertain.

Although thiazide and thiazide-like diuretics are generally well tolerated and can enhance the blood-pressure-lowering effect of other drug classes, they can be associated with several unwanted metabolic effects, including:

- hypokalaemia (drug and dose dependent)
- worsening glucose tolerance (particularly when prescribed in combination with a β-blocker)
- slight worsening of serum lipid profile (rises in LDL-C and triglycerides)
- small rise in serum urate levels (avoid in gout)
- hypercalcaemia.

Thiazide or thiazide-like diuretics can also cause erectile dysfunction. They interact with nonsteroidal anti-inflammatory drugs (less effect on blood pressure lowering) and lithium (increased risk of lithium toxicity). The BNF states that the thiazide-related diuretic indapamide is "claimed to produce less metabolic disturbance", particularly less hyperglycaemia, although hypokalaemia is still possible.

In the large ALLHAT trial (ALLHAT 2002), the thiazide chlorthalidone was found to be as effective as as amlodipine (a DCCB) and lisinopril (an ACE inhibitor) as an initial blood-pressure-lowering therapy for reducing cardiovascular events; also, chlorthalidone reduced heart failure when compared with amlodipine. The INSIGHT trial found no significant difference in the overall onset of cardiovascular events between co-amilozide and the CCB nifedipine (Mancia et al 2003). However, in ALLHAT increased rates of hypokalaemia and increased cholesterol and fasting glucose levels occurred on chlorthalidone, significantly when compared to lisinopril, but of minimal clinical significance when compared to amlodipine. In the ASCOT study, the group in which bendroflumethiazide was used as an add-in drug had a poorer cardiovascular outcome (Dahlöf et al 2006), but how much was this due to the effect of the first-line drug atenolol, the levels of blood pressure achieved or the effects on other cardiovascular risk factors? Nonetheless, thiazide diuretics remain recommended as first line in the 2006 NICE and ADA guidelines.

Loop diuretics are often better than thiazides at augmenting the blood-pressure-lowering effect of ACE inhibitors/ARBs.

Alpha (α)-1 adrenergic blockers

This drug class can be sub-divided into selective (e.g. *doxazosin, indoramin, prazosin* and *terazosin*) and nonselective (*phentolamine*). These drugs block the activation of post-synaptic α-1 adrenoreceptors in the vasculature, resulting in arteriolar and venous vasodilatation. The selective α-1 blockers do not affect glucose tolerance, uric acid and potassium levels; furthermore, they appear to improve lipid profiles by reducing total cholesterol and triglycerides, while increasing HDL-C.

The major side effects of α-1 blockers are first-dose syncope and orthostatic hypotension. These effects can be minimised or prevented by prescribing a low initial dose and by avoiding concomitant prescribing of diuretics. Alpha-1 blockers should be used with caution in the elderly, since their side effects increase the risk of falls. The short-acting prazosin, one of the earlier members of this class, is more likely to cause postural hypotension than the longer-acting doxazosin or terazosin. Other side-effects of α-1 blockers include fatigue, weakness, stuffy nose and headache.

The α-blocker arm of the ALLHAT study used doxazosin and was terminated after an interim analysis showed that doxazosin was significantly less effective than diuretic therapy (chlortalidone) in preventing cardiovascular events (ALLHAT 2000).

These drugs may alleviate the symptoms of benign prostatic hypertrophy in men, particularly if there is detrusor hyperactivity, but can exacerbate stress incontinence in women.

Spironolactone

This potassium-retaining diuretic acts by blocking sodium/potassium exchange in the renal distal tubules. It has two main roles in blood pressure lowering:

1. It may limit potassium loss in patients treated with thiazide or thiazide-like diuretics.
2. Hyperaldosteronism is more common in "resistant" hypertension than previously recognised. Spironolactone can be very effective as a fourth-line drug in patients whose blood pressure levels may be dependent on hyperaldosteronism (Hood et al 2002).

The NICE 2006 guidelines recommend spironolactone as a possible add-in drug in difficult-to-treat hypertension when combinations of the three standard first-line agents have not lowered blood pressure sufficiently. Potassium-retaining diuretics need to be monitored carefully in patients with impaired renal function due to the risk of developing hyperkalaemia, particularly if combined with either an ACE inhibitor or ARB. Spironolactone can commonly cause gynaecomastia due to its anti-androgen effect. A recent population-based, case-control study claimed to find an association between spironolactone and upper gastro-intestinal bleeding and ulcers (Verhamme et al 2006), although there may be confounding factors and causality was not proven.

Centrally acting, older and other antihypertensive agents

Once a mainstay in blood-pressure-lowering treatment, centrally acting, older and other antihypertensive drugs are currently reserved for patients whose raised blood pressure is not controlled by, or who have contraindications to, the other drug classes. These agents are less favoured than other drug groups because side effects can be more frequent, and may be unpleasant or potentially dangerous.

These drugs include:

1. **Sympatholytic agents**, which can be subdivided into:
    *   the imidazoline (I1) agonist, *moxonidine*, which binds highly selectively to imidazoline receptors in the brain's venterolateral medulla, causing reduced peripheral sympathetic activity. This leads to falls in peripheral resistance and blood pressure. Moxonidine has little effect on α-2 receptors, which cause dry mouth and sedation.
    *   the central α-agonists, *methyldopa* and *clonidine*, reduce sympathetic vasoconstriction and total peripheral vascular resistance. The major side effects of these drugs are dose-related: sedation and drowsiness.
2. **The vasodilators**, *hydralazine, diazoxide* and *minoxidil*, act by relaxing vascular smooth muscle, producing decreased peripheral vascular resistance. Their major side effects include gastrointestinal upset and fluid retention. Minoxidil may cause hirsutism, an effect exploited by its topical use in balding men.

Which drugs should be chosen?

When reviewing evidence, it is crucial to distinguish between "surrogate" endpoints of levels of blood pressure achieved and the "real" endpoints of mortality or morbidity. The characteristics and treatments of subjects recruited into drug trials may not resemble those of patients frequently encountered in primary care.

Which drug should be the initial therapy?

As stated above, five drug classes (ACE inhibitors, ARBs, β-blockers, CCBs and diuretics) have been shown to reduce cardiovascular events in individuals with both diabetes and hypertension (ADA 2004, Clinical Evidence online). Which of these drug classes should be the first-line therapy in patients with type 2 diabetes and raised blood pressure? There is no simple answer.

The most recent JBS guidelines concluded that "in general the various drug classes are about as effective as each other at reducing cardiovascular mortality and morbidity per unit fall in blood pressure" ... with the caveat that there is "heterogeneity in response to different drug classes, optimal drug combinations, and specific categories of hypertension" (Wood et al 2005). The ADA recommends initial drug therapy with an agent from one of the five drug classes listed above (ADA 2004). For routine treatment, the 2006 NICE guidelines recommend choosing from ACE inhibitors, ARBs, DCCBs and diuretics, but *not* β-blockers, except in pregnant women or in patients with CHD and/or heart failure (NICE 2006a).

In the 2006 NICE treatment template (see Table 4.7), the reasoning behind drug selection is that hypertension can be classified as "high renin" and "low renin" and, as such, it is best treated initially with drugs that either inhibit the renin-angiotensin system (ACE inhibitor or ARB, known as A drugs) or those that do not inhibit the renin-angiotensin system (CCB or a thiazide diuretic – known as C or D drugs). "Younger" people (aged 55 years or less) tend to have higher renin levels in comparison to older people and blacks of all ages. Thus, the recommended initial therapy in the former group is a drug from the A group, and in the latter group a drug from the C or D group. This is a change from earlier (2004) NICE guidance which stated that there was

TABLE 4.7 The NICE 2006 recommendations for combining blood-pressure-lowering drugs (NICE Clinical Guideline 2006a)

	Younger than 55 years	55 years or older or black patients of any age
	↓	↓
Step 1	A	C or D
	↓	
Step 2	A + C or A + D	
	↓	
Step 3	A + C + D	
	↓	
Step 4 (Resistant hypertension)	Add further diuretic therapy (spironolactone or increase dosage of thiazide) OR α-blocker OR β-blocker	
Step 5 (Failure to respond to 4 drugs)	Referral to specialist clinic	

Key: A = ACE inhibitor or ARB; C = calcium channel blocker; D = diuretic (thiazide)

"no compelling evidence" to support the opinion that different classes of drug are more effective in lowering the risk of developing CVD in either older or younger age patients (North of England Hypertension Guideline Development Group 2004).

In patients with diabetes and incipient or established heart failure, blockade of the renin-angiotensin and of the cardiac sympathetic nervous systems with ACE inhibitors and β-blockers, respectively, improves outcomes. The cardioprotective effects of these drug classes should be taken into consideration when selecting a blood-pressure-lowering agent.

Nevertheless, the reader should bear in mind the findings of three studies:

1. The UKPDS showed that a blood pressure reduction of 10/5 mmHg reduced the incidence of diabetes complications. However, the trial was underpowered to compare the main agents used, captopril and atenolol (UKPDS 1998a).
2. The ALLHAT (antihypertensive and lipid lowering to prevent heart attack trial) study found no large differences between initial therapy with either chlortalidone, lisinopril or amlodipine in reducing blood pressure and cardiovascular events (ALLHAT 2002), notwithstanding certain concerns about the trial's design and conclusions. A further analysis of the ALLHAT results found "no evidence of superiority for treatment with CCB or ACE inhibitors compared with a thiazide-type diuretic during first-step antihypertensive therapy in diabetes mellitus, IFG, or normoglycaemia" (Whelton et al 2005).
3. The Blood Pressure Lowering Treatment Trialists' Collaboration conducted a meta-analysis of 29 trials that involved 162 341 participants with over 700 000 years of follow-up and found that "*the main driver from BP-lowering therapy is BP lowering per se*" (Blood Pressure Lowering Treatment Trialists' Collaboration 2003).

There has been a debate as to whether ethnicity contributes to different outcomes in drug treatments; nevertheless, there is strong evidence that blood-pressure-lowering therapy reduces cardiovascular risk irrespective of ethnicity (ALLHAT 2000). Blood pressure in blacks often responds well to dietary salt restriction and there are theoretical reasons why thiazides and CCBs may be more effective in lowering blood pressure than β-blockers, ACE or ARB. However, a review by the University of York in 2004 (University of York 2004) concluded that "there is insufficient evidence that any antihypertensive drug or drug combination is superior in reducing morbidity and mortality outcomes in hypertensive black people." There is also no evidence currently available to show that South Asians respond differently than white Europeans to blood-pressure-lowering medication. A recent meta-analysis suggested that adverse reactions to cardiovascular drugs, including ACE inhibitors and thrombolytic therapy, may be different between some ethnic groups: a factor that may influence clinical decisions about drug choices and doses (McDowell et al 2006).

Considering all of the above, the following approach seems sensible:

- The first-line agent should be from a drug class that has been shown to reduce CVD events in diabetics.
- Contraindications, potential side-effects, likely tolerability, potential drug interactions and the logistics of monitoring all need to be taken into account when making a choice.

- When heart failure is either incipient or established, blockade of the renin-angiotensin and of the cardiac sympathetic nervous systems with ACE inhibitors and β-blockers, respectively, is desirable.
- When diabetic nephropathy is incipient, established or worsening, ACE inhibitors/ARBs should be considered first.
- Most patients will need combination therapy (see Table 4.7).
- The importance of modifying other cardiovascular risk factors must not be ignored.

The most important message, however, is that:

The extent of blood pressure lowering is probably more important than the choice of agent(s). Even a small reduction in blood pressure will improve outcome.

Combining drug groups rationally

In many patients, more than one blood-pressure-lowering drug needs to be prescribed concurrently to achieve target or produce a substantial reduction in blood pressure. Several factors may influence the selection of the second or third (or even fourth) drug in the combination. These include tolerability, potential drug interactions, and contraindications.

The BHS 2004 Guidelines introduced a treatment template to assist practitioners to combine different drug classes in a rational and effective way. This was modified in the 2006 NICE guidelines, shown in Table 4.7. Ultimately, the aim should be to achieve the best possible blood pressure control, with minimal and tolerable side-effects.

DYSLIPIDAEMIA

RATIONALE

QOF◀
DM16
DM17

An abnormal lipid profile (also called dyslipidaemia) is a major independent risk factor in the development of CHD. Cholesterol and triglycerides do not circulate freely in solution in plasma, but are bound to proteins and are transported as macromolecular complexes, known as lipoproteins; these are classified according to their density, ranging from very-low-density lipoproteins (VLDL) through low-density lipoproteins (LDL), then intermediate-density lipoproteins (IDL) to high-density lipoproteins (HDL). Quantitatively, TG is the "major" lipid group transported in the blood, with 70 to 150 g entering and leaving plasma daily, compared with 1 to 2 g of cholesterol. About 70% of the total cholesterol (TC) in plasma is carried in the LDL fraction and 25% is carried in the HDL fraction.

The combination of elevated levels of LDL with reduced levels of HDL predisposes an individual to the development of arteriosclerosis, regardless of whether diabetes is present. There is a direct and continuous association between total and LDL cholesterol levels in the serum and CVD risk, while serum HDL levels have an inverse correlation with CHD risk (Betteridge 1997). The "hallmark" of obesity is the over-production by the liver of VLDL, which is then converted to LDL and is often associated with elevated levels of triglycerides. LDL levels may also be raised due to defective clearance, which has many causes, including reduced numbers or activity of LDL-receptors. Elevated levels of TG have a major adverse effect upon CHD risk. In contrast, HDL has several anti-atherogenic actions. Low HDL-C increases vulnerablity to the dynamic features of atherogenesis (often mediated by raised LDL-C): these include cholesterol accumulation, inflammation, pro-thrombotic activity, matrix fragilisation and oxidative stress. Cholesterol levels can be affected by both genetic (e.g. familial hyperlipoproteinaemias) and environmental factors, and by the presence of other conditions, such as hypothyroidism and obstructive liver disease. Individuals who migrate from a country with a lower prevalence of CVD to a country with a higher prevalence often alter their eating habits and other behaviours accordingly, resulting in a CVD risk closer to that of their new country's endogenous population.

The lipid profile is frequently "adverse" in patients with impaired glucose tolerance or type 2 diabetes: total cholesterol, LDL-C and triglycerides may be elevated, while HDL-C levels are often lower. Also, HDL-C is often "dysfunctional" or less active in patients with diabetes. This abnormal profile often precedes the onset of intermediate hyperglycaemia or diabetes by several years, so that atherogenesis may occur prior to the development of hyperglycaemia.

There is now strong evidence that improving the lipid profile, particularly in lowering LDL-C, does reduce significantly the incidence of CHD mortality and morbidity in individuals at higher risk (Baigent et al 2005).

TARGETS

The aim of lipid modification should be to both improve and maintain lipid levels beyond the threshold at which there is no increased CHD risk. However, there is now evidence that lowering total and LDL-C in high-risk patients (including diabetics), irrespective of the baseline, improves outcomes. For these individuals, the consensus is now moving away from the target being a fixed endpoint to a percentage reduction. This is consistent with the latest guidance from both the Joint British Societies and the ADA, which recommend targets that are either a fixed end point or a minimum percentage reduction, **whichever is lower.**

The range of targets recommended by these and other authoritative bodies is summarised in Table 4.8. The current national policy (NICE and NSF) for lipid targets (whichever results in a lower absolute level) is a total cholesterol less than 5.0 mmol/l (or reduced by 20–25%), and a LDL-C less than 3.0 mmol/l (or reduced by 30%), instead of JBS2's lower recommended optimal levels. However, these targets may be revised when NICE issues its guidance on lipid modification (at writing, due December 2007). As with other risk factors, it is sensible to set less strict targets in some older patients with a limited life expectancy.

The latest JBS2 guidelines do not give targets for either triglyceride or HDL-C, due to a lack of evidence from interventional studies.

The ADA's recommended targets do not include total cholesterol, only lipoprotein functions. In addition to LDL-C, the ADA targets, in diabetics **with overt CVD**, include:

- Triglyceride levels less than 1.7 mmol/l
- HDL-C levels greater than 1.15 mmol/l in men and 1.44 mmol/l in women (ADA 2007).

TABLE 4.8 Target lipid levels recommended by different learned bodies or organisations

Total cholesterol target (mmol/l) whichever is lower	LDL-C target (mmol/l) whichever is lower	Learned body/ organisation	Date published
<5.0 in "high risk"	Not stated	SIGN	November 2001
<5.0 (or 20–25% reduction)	<3.0 (or 30% reduction)	NICE/NSF	2000
Not stated	<2.6 or 30–40% reduction	ADA	January 2006
<5.0 "audit standard"	<3.0 "audit standard"	JBS 2	December 2005
<4.0 "optimal" or 25% reduction	<2.0 "optimal" or 30% reduction		

The new GMS contract QOF's only current lipid target is a total cholesterol of less than 5.0 mmol/l, although this could change in the future. Looking at the most recent evidence, simply achieving this target may not correct an atherogenic lipid profile sufficiently, especially in high-risk patients. Primary care teams should consider setting a target for LDL-C, and possibly HDL-C and triglycerides, in high-risk patients.

Future recommendations are likely to demand an even more "aggressive" approach to lipid regulation, where there would be *no lower limit* for intervention in or for the target of LDL-C in high-risk patients.

EVALUATION

Serum lipid estimation is best done after an overnight fast, because chylomicrons from the last meal can affect triglyceride levels. The practice should request that the local chemical pathology laboratory provides total cholesterol, lipoprotein fractions, and triglyceride levels in its report. Most laboratories will give LDL-C and HDL-C values.

INTERVENTIONS: OVERVIEW

The management of dyslipidaemia can be divided into pharmacological and nonpharmacological methods. Irrespective of the baseline levels, improving the lipid profile will reduce cardiovascular risk in all type 2 diabetics.

INTERVENTIONS: NONPHARMACOLOGICAL

Nonpharmacological management should not be overlooked. Weight loss, reduced alcohol intake and increased levels of physical activity can lead to decreased TG and LDL cholesterol, and increased HDL levels (behavioural change is currently the most effective way of raising HDL-C levels). Improved glycaemic control will lower TG levels. "Maximal" dietary modification can reduce LDL cholesterol by up to 0.65 mmol/l.

Unless the patient is at high risk requiring immediate drug treatment, a trial period of from 3 to 6 months is useful to ascertain the success of a dietary and/or exercise regimen.

INTERVENTIONS: PHARMACOLOGICAL MANAGEMENT

There are several classes of lipid-regulating drugs currently available. The statins are the mainstay of lipid-regulating pharmacotherapy, but it is both important and useful to know about the other classes of lipid-regulating drugs.

In support of the Diabetes NSF, the National Clinical Guidelines for Type 2 Diabetes published its recommendations in 2002 for the management of "abnormal" serum lipids (McIntosh et al 2002). Following the findings of several important studies, this guidance has now been superseded by the JBS 2 guidelines published in December 2005:

1. All diabetics should be regarded as being high risk of developing a CVD event.
2. Treatment with a statin is now recommended for all diabetics, with the exception of those under 40 whose most recent HbA1c is not greater than 9.0%, whose total cholesterol is below 6.0 mmol/l, and are without any target organ damage or significant cardiovascular risk factors (these exclusions are likely to disappear, as it is clear that *all* diabetics benefit from LDL-C lowering). Statin treatment is indicated in all those aged under 40 with existing CVD, irrespective of whether diabetes co-exists.
3. Other classes of lipid-regulating drugs should be considered in addition to a statin if the total and LDL cholesterol targets are not achieved, or if levels of HDL-C and/or triglycerides need to be modified.

The American Diabetes Association's 2006 recommendations are quite similar to JBS 2:

1. All those with overt CVD should be treated with a statin to achieve an LDL-C reduction of 30 to 40%.
2. In those without overt CVD:
   a. Treat all those aged 40 years or more with a statin, regardless of baseline LDL-C, to same target
   b. Treat those under the age of 40 years, but at increased risk due to other cardiovascular risk factors, and not achieving lipid goals with nonpharmacological interventions.

Once started on treatment, patients require earlier review to monitor the response to and the safety of their treatment. A combination of lipid-regulating drugs may be required in high-risk individuals who require aggressive correction of their dyslipidaemia. There are little data available on the reduction in cardiovascular events in patients on combinations of a statin and either a fibrate or nicotinic acid.

A meta-analysis of 12 RCTs (including ALLHAT, ASCOT, MRC/HPS, 4S, LIPID, CARE) comparing the efficacy of lipid-lowering treatment for diabetic and nondiabetic patients, concluded that:

1. Treatment, particularly with statins significantly reduced cardiovascular risk in both diabetic and nondiabetic patients
2. Diabetic patients benefit more than nondiabetic patients from treatment in both primary and secondary prevention, when the results are adjusted for baseline risk (Costa et al 2006).

Although this meta-analysis has some limitations (varying definitions of diabetes, three studies combined results for coronary events and stroke, two studies used gemfibrozil, effects of dose were not explored), it was published after JBS2 and may have important implications for clinical practice: probably "all" patients with type 2 diabetes should receive statin treatment if their LDL-C is equal to or greater than 2.0 mmol/l (Reckless 2006), going beyond the JBS 2 guidelines discussed above.

Statins

Hydroxymethyl glutaryl coenzyme A (HMG-CoA) reductase inhibitors are commonly known as statins and have been available for at least 15 years. By competitive inhibition of the rate-limiting enzyme responsible for the hepatic synthesis of cholesterol, statins block the endogenous synthesis of cholesterol, causing the hepatocyte's cholesterol requirements to be met by the uptake of circulating cholesterol via a catabolic LDL receptor on the cell surface; the number of these receptors is thought to be increased by statins. Statins can reduce plasma LDL-C by up to 40%. These drugs also have a moderate effect on increasing HDL-C and lowering plasma TG levels, although this is less than their effect on LDL-C.

Although statins are usually well tolerated, they should be used with caution in patients with a history of liver disease or with a high alcohol intake. As with fibrates, rhabdomyolysis and reversible myositis are rare but significant side effects of statins, particularly in patients with renal impairment and hypothyroidism or taking concurrent fibrates or ciclosporin. Patients taking statins should have liver function tests (LFTs) and creatine kinase (CK) estimations two to three months after starting treatment, after a further increase in dose, or if symptoms of myositis occur at any time on therapy. They should also be advised to report promptly unexplained muscle pain, tenderness or weakness.

Five statins are currently available in the UK: atorvastatin, *fluvastatin, pravastatin, rosuvastatin* and *simvastatin*. Another statin, *cerivastatin*, was withdrawn due to the risk of rhabdomyolysis when it was used in combination with gemfibrozil (a fibrate).

Several well-publicised trials demonstrated that pravastatin (CARE [Goldberg et al 1998], LIPID 1998, PROSPER [Shepherd et al 2002], WOSCOPS 1998) and simvastatin (Scandinavian Simvastatin Survival Study and MRC/BHF) reduced both total and LDL cholesterol levels and were effective in the primary and secondary prevention of CHD, although the cholesterol levels achieved in many patients in these studies fell short of the JBS 2 targets. In elderly individuals at high risk of developing vascular disease, pravastatin reduced the risk of CHD after 3 years (Shepherd et al 2002). Three recent studies have provided the strongest evidence base for the benefits of lipid lowering using statins in type 2 diabetics:

1. MRC/BHF Heart Protection Study reported that a lowering of LDL-C by 30% (using simvastatin) significantly reduced the risk of a major CHD event at 4.8 years (relative risk reduction 22%, number needed to treat 20), independent of the diabetic patient's baseline LDL-cholesterol (Heart Protection Study Collaborative Group 2003).
2. In 2004 the Collaborative AtoRvastatin Diabetes Study (CARDS) recruited 2838 type 2 diabetics. It reported that, compared with placebo, treatment with atorvastatin 10 mg significantly reduced cardiovascular events at 3.9 years (absolute risk reduction 3.2%, RRR 35.6%, NNT 32). Acute coronary events were reduced by 36%, coronary revascularisation by 31% and stroke by 48% in the atorvastatin group. Baseline lipids, sex and age did not affect the results (Colhoun et al 2004).
3. The ASCOT primary prevention trial of high-risk, uncontrolled hypertensive patients recruited 2532 patients with diabetes. In the lipid-lowering arm, subjects had a baseline nonfasting TC below 6.5 mmol/l. The primary endpoint of nonfatal MI plus fatal CHD was reduced by over one-third more in patients treated with atorvastatin 10 mg compared to placebo, even with equivalent blood pressure reduction (Sever et al 2003).

Furthermore, a meta-analysis of 14 RCTs concluded that an absolute reduction in LDL-C, independently of the baseline level, reduces CVD risk (relative risk reduction of 21% in CVD events per mmol/l reduction in LDL-C). This effect appears to apply equally to subgroups in which there had been previous uncertainty, such as people with diabetes and no pre-existing vascular disease and people aged more than 75 years (Baigent et al 2005).

Although, in its 2006 technology appraisal of statins, NICE accepted that statin therapy is "cost-effective" in type 2 diabetics, it concluded "that the decision whether to initiate statin therapy in diabetics should be made where a clinical assessment has estimated the CVD risk to be likely to be equivalent to at least 20% over 10 years." Since NICE noted that there were "no data on clinical events to suggest the superiority of any one statin over all the others in reducing cardiovascular events", it recommended initial statin therapy using "a drug with low acquisition cost" (NICE 2006b).

Some of NICE's conclusions may seem a little surprising as:

1. By introducing an assessment of CVD risk for this population (despite noting the "limitations of assessing risk in diabetics using standard risk calculators"!), NICE infers that not all patients with diabetes are at high risk, a standpoint not supported by a wide range of evidence.
2. NICE contradicts the most recent authoritative guidance given by both the Joint British Societies and the ADA.

3. Cardiovascular risk is reduced in all diabetics on statin therapy that lowers total cholesterol and LDL-C levels, irrespective of baseline lipid profile.

A "new generation" synthetic statin, *rosuvastatin*, is more potent than other statins in lowering LDL-C levels (achieving up to 45–50% reduction). In the ASTEROID study patients with existing atheroma were all prescribed maximal dose (40 mg) rosuvastatin for 2 years. Not only did a significantly better lipid profile (lower LDL-C and higher HDL-C) result, but a "significant" median reduction in fatty deposits occurred, suggesting that the treatment produced a regression in the build up of fatty deposits in the coronary arteries (Nissen et al 2006). Due to lack of controls on a lower dose of rosuvastatin or on a high dose of another statin, and the relatively short duration of this study, further research is needed to answer the following important questions:

• Do these changes lead to improved clinical outcomes?
• Are these changes dose-related?
• Would other statins have produced a similar effect?

ASTEROID reported "infrequent" side-effects, despite previous reports of increased risk of serious muscle toxicity associated with rosuvastatin, particularly in certain subpopulations (renal impairment, hypothyroidism, Japanese and Chinese origin, alcohol abuse, concomitant use of fibrates) to the US Food and Drug Administration (FDA) and other regulatory bodies. These led to revised guidance being issued in 2004 for prescribing rosuvastatin, advising that mainly the lower doses of 5–10 mg should be prescribed in primary care, with the maximum dose of 40 mg to be prescribed only under close (i.e. specialist) supervision and with greater caution. NICE indicated that, particularly with insufficient data on clinical events currently available for rosuvastatin, there is "significant uncertainty" over rosuvastatin's cost-effectiveness (NICE 2006b). Currently, rosuvastatin is a second-line drug, but it may be increasingly used when "older" statins fail to achieve the progressively "tighter" targets set by authoritative bodies.

A note of caution should be introduced at this point. Statins do not produce significant increases in low HDL-C levels. Women and non-Caucasians were not always well represented in lipid-lowering interventional studies and currently there are no published studies reporting the effect of lipid-lowering therapy on "hard" cardiovascular outcomes in any population originating from the Indian subcontinent (Winocour and Fisher 2003). Being a female and/or nonwhite diabetic does increase an individual's susceptibility to the adverse effects of many cardiovascular risk factors. However, it is reasonable, until further evidence is published, not to allow the patient's gender or ethnicity to influence decisions about the type of therapy to reduce cardiovascular risk.

"At the end of the day" while there may be some subgroups of type 2 diabetics in whom the evidence for the benefits of statin therapy may be considered less robust than in others (Drugs and Therapeutics Bulletin 2006), there is a clear consensus in the guidance from JBS2 and the ADA: all type 2 diabetics aged over 40 (and many aged under 40) are at increased CVD risk, regardless of baseline levels, and should be on a statin.

Anion-exchange resins (bile acid sequestrants)

The two available agents in this drug class are *cholestyramine* and *colestipol*. They act by binding bile acids in the gut, preventing their re-absorption. This promotes conversion of cholesterol into bile acids by the liver, resulting in increased LDL-receptor activity of hepatic cells which increases LDL-cholesterol clearance. Also, since bile acids are required for the intestinal absorption of sterols, use of these agents results in increased faecal loss of dietary cholesterol. Although these drugs reduce LDL-cholesterol by up to 25% more than by dietary modification alone, they can aggravate hypertriglyceridaemia.

Anion-exchange resins are not especially palatable. They are not absorbed and can cause gastro-intestinal side-effects (constipation more than diarrhoea, nausea, vomiting and discomfort) and can interfere with the absorption of fat-soluble vitamins (A, D and K – supplementation may be necessary on long-term therapy).

Currently there are no systematic reviews or RCTs in people with diabetes and higher risk for macrovascular complications comparing anion exchange resins (colestyramine, colestipol) versus placebo or comparisons of different anion exchange resins, or different doses for CVD outcomes.

Fibrates

Fibrates are broad-spectrum, lipid-modulating agents. Their use can lead to:

- Decreased serum TG levels
- A reduction of LDL-C by up to 18%
- Increased HDL-C levels
- Decreased VLDL levels.

The currently available fibrates are bezafibrate, ciprofibrate, fenofibrate and gemfibrozil.

All fibrates can cause rhabdomyolysis or other muscle toxicities. These usually present as muscle pain, associated with elevated serum creatine phosphokinase (CPK), particularly in patients with impaired renal function or hypothyroidism. The risk of muscle toxicity is increased if a fibrate is taken concurrently with a statin or ciclosporin. There is also a risk of a rise in serum creatinine, particularly with fenofibrate.

Bezafibrate suppresses endogenous synthesis of cholesterol and triglycerides. It also "causes the expression" of an increased number of specific LDL receptors, increasing the catabolism of LDL-C. Triglyceride catabolism is stimulated through systemic lipoprotein lipase and hepatic lipase. Ciprofibrate and fenofibrate lower plasma LDL, VLDL and TG levels and raise serum HDL levels without increasing the risk of developing gall stones. Gemfibrozil reduces raised levels of TG, TC, LDL-C and VLDL and raises low levels of HDL-C. Its lowering of plasma TG levels is likely to be achieved by reducing the hepatic synthesis of VLDL and increasing VLDL clearance.

Five randomised controlled trials (RCTs) found that fibrates, compared to placebo, have a "beneficial effect" upon cardiovascular mortality and morbidity and improve triglyceride levels (Clinical Evidence online). However, questions over safety were raised in two primary prevention studies (Koskinen et al 1992), while two secondary prevention studies suggested that fibrates were quite safe (Heinonen 1994, Rubins et al 1999).

The Fenofibrate Intervention and Event Lowering in Diabetes (FIELD) trial, comparing treatment with fenofibrate against placebo, provided mixed results. Fenofibrate did not significantly reduce the risk of the primary trial outcome of major coronary events. However, in the group treated with fenofibrate, there were fewer total cardiovascular disease events and a significant reduction in microvascular-associated complications. Fenobrate appeared also to be generally well tolerated in type 2 diabetics (Keech et al 2005).

Since statins are less effective in raising low HDL-C, alternative drug classes (such as fibrates and nicotinic acid group) need to be considered in lipid management. Despite the problems associated with combining gemfibrozil and the withdrawn statin cerivastatin, the need to raise HDL-C levels, along with lowering LDL-C and TG levels, may prompt the clinician to consider prescribing a statin–fibrate combination. Compared with fluvastatin plus placebo, fluvastatin plus fenofibrate significantly improved lipid profile in people with type 2 diabetes, dyslipidaemia, and history of CHD (Derosa et al 2004). It appears that this combination is relatively well tolerated, provided that renal, hepatic and thyroid function remains normal with CPK levels being monitored and that any muscle pains are promptly reported.

Cholesterol absorption inhibitors

This drug group selectively inhibits cholesterol transport across the wall of the small intestine, thus reducing the delivery of intestinal cholesterol to the liver. *Ezetimibe* is the first available product in this class. It is metabolised in the liver and small intestine to its active glucuronide form, which undergoes enterohepatic recycling, prolonging its action. Ezetimibe is not a bile acid sequestrant. It does not interfere with the absorption of TG, fatty acids or fat-soluble vitamins. Headache, abdominal pain and diarrhoea are common side effects of ezetimibe.

Ezetimibe's licenses include:

- Adjunctive therapy to dietary modification in patients with hypercholesterolaemia, either in combination with a statin (acting synergistically to lower LDL-C levels) or as monotherapy (if a statin is inappropriate or contraindicated).
- Treatment of homozygous familial hypercholesterolaemia in combination with dietary modification and a statin.

There are no systematic reviews or RCTs in people with diabetes and higher risk for macrovascular complications comparing ezetimibe versus placebo, or comparisons of different doses for CVD outcomes (Clinical Evidence online). However, compared with statin plus placebo, statin plus ezetimibe significantly improved the lipid profile in type 2 diabetics over 8 weeks (Simons et al 2004). Adding ezetimibe to a statin is much more expensive than maximising the dosage of the statin. When aggressive LDL-C lowering is required, ezetimibe may have a role: either in combination with a statin beyond a maximal statin dose or as an alternative if statins are contraindicated or not tolerated. At the time of writing, NICE plans to issue a technology appraisal of ezetimibe in 2007.

Nicotinic acid group

The nicotinic acid group (*nicotinic acid* and *acipimox* are the currently available drugs in the UK) of drugs improve both serum cholesterol and triglyceride levels.

They appear to act in several ways, including partial inhibition of free fatty acid release from adipose tissue, increased lipoprotein lipase activity and decreased hepatic synthesis of LDL-C; thus producing lower LDL-C and triglyceride levels. Nicotinic acid was reported to increase HDL-C levels significantly in one RCT. However, a large proportion of this study's subjects were also taking a statin (Grundy et al 2002). Nicotinic acid's side effects, especially vasodilatation, can be troublesome. It also worsens glucose tolerance (it may precipitate diabetes).

Nicotinic acid is now available also in an extended-release formulation (Niaspan). Patients started on niaspan may experience transient facial flushing. This drug has been associated with hepatic toxicity; thus, liver function should be monitored prior and during prescribing. Niaspan should be used with caution in patients with a history of liver disease or who consume large quantities of alcohol.

In 2004 the Scottish Medicines Consortium advised that Niaspan was not recommended for the treatment of hypercholesterolaemia and mixed hyperlipidaemia, due to the lack of suitable studies (available at the time) comparing it with other lipid-regulating drugs. However, as with fibrates, the need for aggressive lipid regulation (especially if seeking to raise HDL-C levels and lower TG levels, as well as lowering LDL-C levels) may prompt clinicians to consider prescribing nicotinic acid, particularly in combination with a statin, subject to the cautions stated above.

Acipimox has fewer side effects than nicotinic acid, but may be less effective.

Fish oils

Fish oils reduce serum triglycerides. There are two preparations currently available:

1. Omega-3-acid ethyl esters (Omacor).
2. Omega-3 marine triglycerides (Maxepa). This can sometimes aggravate hypercholesterolaemia.

Increased consumption of fish oils has been recommended for some time, as this was said to be linked with a number of positive health outcomes, including protection from cardiovascular disease (Brunner 2006). However, a recent systematic review concluded that "long chain and shorter chain omega 3 fats do not have a clear effect on total mortality, combined cardiovascular events, or cancer" (Hooper et al 2006).

Selection of drug therapy

Five classes of lipid-modifying drugs (but not all drugs within each class) have been shown in clinical trials to reduce myocardial infarction and coronary death: statins, fibrates, anion exchange resins, nicotinic acid and its derivatives, and fish oils. However, the largest and most convincing body of clinical trial data is for the use of a statin in reducing CVD and total mortality.

Table 4.9 summarises the indications, cautions and contraindications relating to the different classes of lipid-modifying drugs.

TABLE 4.9 Compelling and possible indications, contraindications and cautions for the major classes of lipid-modifying drugs (Wood et al 2005)

Class of drug	Compelling indications	Possible indications	Cautions	Compelling contraindications

Statins	1. Atherosclerotic CVD
	2. DM
	  a. all aged ≥40
	  b. 18–39 with compelling indications
	3. CVD 10-year risk ≥20%
	4. Familial hypercholesterolaemia
		CVD 10-year risk 10–20% if either: TC/HDL ratio >6 or LDL-C > 5 mmol/l	1. Non-alcoholic steatohepatitis
			2. Untreated hypothyroidism
			3. Significant chronic renal impairment (creatinine > 160 mmol/l)
			4. Some drugs metabolised through cytochrome P450
			5. Excess alcohol intake
			6. Grapefruit juice consumed in large quantities
				1. Gemfibrozil
				2. Significant liver disease

Fibrates	1. Type III hypercholesterolaemia 2. Severe hypertriglyceridaemia	1. Type 2 DM with raised TG and low HDL-C 2. Moderate–severe hypertriglyceridaemia with controlled LDL-C	1. Chronic renal failure 2. Concurrent statin therapy	Never use gemfibrozil with a statin
Anion exchange resins	None (poor GI tolerability)	1. Inadequate LDL-C control on statin-ezetimibe combination 2. Cholestasis with itching	1. GI upset 2. Exacerbation of hypertriglyceridaemia 3. Interaction with other drugs 4. Reduction in fat-soluble vitamin absorption	None

Continued

TABLE 4.9 Compelling and possible indications, contraindications and cautions for the major classes of lipid-modifying drugs (Wood et al 2005)—Cont'd

Class of drug	Compelling indications	Possible indications	Cautions	Compelling contraindications
Nicotinic acid group	1. Severe hypertriglyceridaemia with prior acute pancreatitis 2. Type V (severe hypertriglyceridaemia not responsive to fibrates)	In combination with other lipid-modifying drugs (most often used in mixed hyperlipidaemia)	1. Other lipid-modifying drugs 2. Impaired renal function 3. Liver disease 4. Diabetes melitus 5. Gout 6. Peptic ulcer 7. Flushing, diarrhoea as side effects	1. Worsening glucose intolerance 2. Diarrhoea and/or flushing
Cholesterol absorption inhibitors	Familial sitosterolaemia	1. With a statin if LDL-C target not reached 2. Statin intolerance	1. Liver impairment 2. With fibrates	None
Fish oils	1. Severe hypertriglyceridaemia 2. CHD prevention	Treatment of hypertriglyceridaemia		None

If target lipid levels are not achieved with the first-line drug, then the following need to be considered:

1. Switching to more potent drugs (usually a second-generation statin)
2. Adding in ezetimibe or fibrate
3. Consider and correct, where appropriate, secondary causes, e.g. hypothyroidism, abnormal liver function
4. Improve glycaemic control (lowers serum TG and raises serum HDL-C)
5. Referral to either a lipid clinic or a diabetic clinic if all else fails or if the medication used causes problems.

Future possible approaches to lipid regulation

With the availability and proven effectiveness of LDL-C-lowering therapies, the future emphasis of drug development and of trials will undoubtedly move towards HDL-C-raising interventions.

OBESITY

DEFINITIONS AND TERMINOLOGY

QOF ◄
DM2
OB1

The World Health Organization (WHO) defines obesity as "a disease state in which excess fat has accumulated to an extent that health may be adversely affected." The WHO categorises body weight into: normal weight, overweight, obesity and severe obesity, using the body mass index (BMI), expressed as kg/m^2. NICE defines "morbid" obesity as greater than $40 kg/m^2$ or between 35 and $40 kg/m^2$ with other significant disease (e.g. diabetes, hypertension) (NICE 2002).

RATIONALE

Obesity with an abdominal distribution (also known as central obesity), rather with gluteal fat accumulation, is associated with metabolic syndrome, insulin resistance and a higher cardiovascular risk (particularly through dyslipidaemia), although it has not yet been demonstrated that obesity is an independent cardiovascular risk factor in diabetes.

Excess weight is almost always due to an imbalance between physical activity and dietary calorific intake: too little of the former in relation to too much of the latter. Any intervention to produce weight loss must correct this imbalance.

From a public health perspective, obesity is becoming an "epidemic", contributing to the relentlessly rising prevalence of metabolic syndrome and diabetes. In England 66% of men and 55% of women are classified as either overweight or obese (Department of Health 2004). The Department of Health has issued guidance available on its website (DoH 2006).

TARGETS

Achieving and maintaining an ideal body weight does not invariably equate with abolishing obesity. Depending upon the definition of obesity, the suggested targets are:

- The ideal *BMI* is greater than $20\,kg/m^2$ and less than $25\,kg/m^2$ in whites ($23\,kg/m^2$ in Indo-Asians).
- The ideal *waist circumference* is less than 102 cm in white men, 88 cm in white women, 90 cm in Asian-Pacific men and 80 cm in Asian-Pacific women.

Substantial and sustained weight loss is not easy to achieve. It is both practical and humane, particularly as the loss has to result mainly from behavioural change, to set a target whose end point takes into account the starting point and that does not require an excessive rate of loss (no more than 1 to 2 kg per month). As patients get older, weight loss becomes progressively more difficult. A realistic target in some individuals may be simply to avoid further weight gain.

EVALUATION

To calculate body mass index (BMI), the height and weight of the patient need to be measured. The calculation, usually done automatically when the data are entered onto a software system, is:

BMI = weight (in kilograms) divided by the square of height (in metres).

BMI is a measure of body *weight* and not of body fat or its distribution, whereas obesity indicates the presence of excessive fat, but not necessarily of excessive body weight: BMI and weight are not measures of the same thing. Some diabetics have increased intra-abdominal fat, but a normal range BMI. The BMI ranges used in most risk tables are characteristic of a white population.

Measuring skin-fold thickness can under-estimate body fat in individuals with mainly central obesity instead of gluteal fat accumulation. Although the waist–hip ratio (WHR) can be calculated, it may underestimate intra-abdominal obesity if gluteal obesity is also present.

The waist circumference is measured half way between the lowest point of the rib cage and the iliac crest (Despres & Lemieur 2001). It is an essential criterion for the diagnosis of metabolic syndrome, and a better predictor than BMI of cardiovascular and metabolic risk. In 2003 Diabetes UK produced a stratification of co-morbidity risk, correlated with BMI and waist circumference in adults, summarised in Table 4.10.

INTERVENTIONS

As with other risk factors, the most important component in the management of obesity is changing the patient's behaviour. The imbalance between an excessive dietary calorific intake and an inadequate level of physical activity needs to be reversed. The

TABLE 4.10 Co-morbidity risks associated with different levels of BMI and waist circumference (from Diabetes UK – Connor et al 2003)

	Caucasian		Asian-Pacific	
	Waist circumference (cm)		Waist circumference (cm)	
Male	<102	≥102	<90	≥90
Female	<88	≥88	<80	≥80
Risk of co-morbidity	BMI	BMI	BMI	BMI
Low (but ↑ other risks)	<18.5		<18.5	
Average	18.5–24.9	<18.5	18.5–22.9	<18.5
Increased	25.0–29.9	18.5–24.9	23.0–24.9	18.5–22.9
Moderate	30.0–34.9	25.0–29.9	25.0–29.9	23.0–24.9
Severe	35.0–39.9	30.0–34.9	30.0–34.9	25.0–29.9
Very severe	≥40.0	≥35.0	≥35.0	≥30.0

target weight and rate of loss should be negotiated. When weight loss is an important on-going activity for the patient, more frequent reviews may be needed to monitor progress and to encourage the patient. Specialist help should be sought if the patient is very obese or fails to respond to medical interventions.

Anti-obesity drugs

Anti-obesity agents may help diabetics to lose weight when prescribed in combination with a restricted energy diet and, ideally, increased physical activity. There are three agents in current use, which act by different mechanisms. *Orlistat* and *sibutramine* have been shown to produce clinically significant weight loss in type 2 diabetics, including those treated with sulphonylureas. All three drugs are expensive.

1. **Orlistat** (proprietary name Xenical) acts within the stomach and small intestine as a long-acting inhibitor of pancreatic lipases. Its mode of action is to prevent the hydrolysis and subsequent absorption of ingested dietary fat (about 30%). The current prescribing licence for orlistat allows it to be prescribed to diabetics aged 18 to 75 years with a BMI of $28 \, kg/m^2$ or more, who can adhere to a hypocaloric diet. Treatment with orlistat can be continued up to 12 months (occasionally up to 24 months), provided that a further 5% of body weight is lost by the end of 3 months' treatment. The decision to continue orlistat for longer than 12 months (usually for weight maintenance) should be made after considering the potential benefits and limitations with the patient (NICE 2006c).

2. **Sibutramine** (proprietary name Reductil) is an anorectic agent that acts centrally by inhibiting serotonin and norepinephrine reuptake, resulting in enhanced satiety. Patients will feel satisfied with smaller food portions. Sibutramine has several important contraindications (important macro- and microvascular disease, uncontrolled hypertension, severe renal impairment, glaucoma, benign prostatic hypertrophy with urinary retention) and it interacts with a number of other drugs, including antidepressants, drugs affecting CYP3A4 or serotonin levels. Sibutramine can be prescribed to diabetics aged 18 to 65 years with a BMI of 27kg/m^2 or more. Continuation beyond the first 4 weeks requires a weight loss of 2 kg; while continuation beyond 3 months requires a loss of 5% of the initial weight at the start of treatment. The maximum duration of treatment in the licence is 12 months (NICE 2006c).

3. **Rimonabant** (proprietary name Acomplia) received its European Union licence in June 2006, but has not gained approval in the US. It is the first in a new class of drugs that selectively inhibits the endocannabinoid system, which plays an important role in the control of appetite, as well as regulating pleasure, relaxation and pain tolerance. Rimonabant is indicated as an adjunct to diet and exercise in obese patients with a BMI equal to or greater than 30kg/m^2 or in overweight patients with a BMI greater than 27kg/m^2 and associated risk factors such as type 2 diabetes or dyslipidaemia. Reports from phase 3 trials show that the use of the drug resulted in improvements in several cardiovascular risk factors (weight loss, reduction in waist circumference, reduced triglycerides and increased HDL-C), as well as reductions in fasting plasma glucose (Van Gaal et al 2005, Pi-Sunyer et al 2006). However, one in eight study subjects at the higher 20 mg dose discontinued medication, most commonly due to gastro-intestinal side effects or depression; other adverse effects include upper respiratory tract infections, headache and dizziness. Rimonabant's efficacy and safety has not been evaluated beyond two years. Based upon the relevant studies excluding subjects with psychiatric disorders and reporting an increased number of adverse psychiatric events, rimonabant is not recommended for patients with significant psychiatric disease or an antidepressant medication. Prescription is best initiated only under specialist supervision. Although rimonabant also shows promise in assisting smoking cessation, further data are required before it gains approval for this indication. The drug's long-term effects, particularly on the endocannabinoid system (with its widespread receptors), also need further evaluation.

Gastric reduction (bariatric) surgery

The use of surgery to limit food intake and produce long-term weight loss is a radical and costly approach to reduce obesity. Several surgical techniques are now available. These include jejuno-ileal bypass, vertical banded gastroplasty and gastric bypass, all of which can result in significant weight loss. The more invasive the surgery, the greater the associated mortality and morbidity, but continuing or worsening severe obesity also carries significant risk to the patient of medical complications.

In the NICE 2006 guidance, "bariatric surgery is recommended as a treatment option for adults with obesity if all of the following criteria are fulfilled:

- they have a BMI of 40 kg/m^2 or more, or between 35 kg/m^2 and 40 kg/m^2 and other significant disease (for example, type 2 diabetes or high blood pressure) that could be improved if they lost weight
- all appropriate non-surgical measures have been tried but have failed to achieve or maintain adequate, clinically beneficial weight loss for at least 6 months
- the person has been receiving or will receive intensive management in a specialist obesity service
- the person is generally fit for anaesthesia and surgery
- the person commits to the need for long-term follow-up."

In addition, NICE recommended bariatric surgery "as a first-line option (instead of lifestyle interventions or drug treatment) for adults with a BMI of more than 50 kg/m^2 in whom surgical intervention is considered appropriate" (Ref NICE 2006c).

NICE did not recommend any particular type of surgery to aid weight loss. The choice of surgical treatment should be made jointly by the individual and the doctor, taking into account individual factors (NICE 2002). Regional centres are now carrying out surgery on a regular basis.

Gastric reduction can be performed *laparoscopically* (using an adjustable LAP-BAND) in which the functional capacity of the stomach is permanently reduced by partitioning off of a small segment of the body of the stomach. This results in a reduced food intake, producing substantial and sustained weight loss in patients with a BMI greater than 35 kg/m^2. It does appear to improve some of the major cardiovascular risk factors (Campbell & Rössner 2001), but there are no current data to compare the long-term benefits and risks of surgery with medical management in diabetics. In a severely obese nondiabetic population, the Swedish Obese Subjects Study reported improvements in lifestyle (lower energy intake and increased physical activity), hypertension and some biochemical variables (lower triglycerides and uric acid, but not hypercholesterolaemia) in those who underwent gastric surgery, compared to those who received conventional medical treatment (Sjöström et al 2004). Technically, this procedure may be difficult or impossible in patients whose BMI is very large (such as greater than 55 kg/m^2), where gastric bypass is preferable.

The older surgical techniques bypass the stomach surgically; thus, restricting the stomach's capacity as well as producing malabsorption. Post-operatively, patients undergoing this type of surgery require permanent vitamin and nutrient supplementation.

REDUCING PLATELET ADHESIVENESS

RATIONALE

Platelets are involved in the development of atherosclerosis and vascular thrombosis. *In vitro* evidence suggests that diabetics are often more sensitive to platelet-aggregating agents. Thromboxane is a potent vasoconstrictor and platelet aggregator. In patients with type 2 diabetes and cardiovascular disease, thromboxane production is increased. Aspirin blocks thromboxane synthesis by acetylating platelet cyclo-oxygenase.

There is considerable evidence from trials and meta-analyses that low-dose aspirin (75–162 mg/day, as effective as and possibly less risky than higher doses) should be prescribed, unless contraindicated, for secondary prevention of cardiovascular events in patients without or with diabetes mellitus. Despite the fact that diabetics with no previous cardiovascular disease run a similarly raised cardiovascular risk to nondiabetics with previous cardiovascular disease, aspirin is under-prescribed in diabetics (ADA Aspirin 2004); however, no studies have been yet published looking at primary prevention of CVD in diabetics using aspirin.

The major risks of aspirin therapy are damage to the gastric mucosa and gastro-intestinal haemorrhage, even at relatively low doses. There is also an increased risk of minor bleeding episodes, such as epistaxis and bruising, but not retinal or vitreous haemorrhage. Enteric-coated preparations do not appear to reduce this risk. The contraindications to prescribing aspirin are allergy, bleeding tendency, concurrent anticoagulation treatment, recent gastro-intestinal haemorrhage, history of asthma triggered by asthma, uncontrolled hypertension, and clinically active hepatic disease.

Clopidogrel (75 mg) may be considered as an alternative to aspirin in patients allergic to aspirin. It is also rather more expensive. There are limited data in diabetics, but one large study found clopidogrel to be slightly more effective than 325 mg aspirin in reducing the combined risk of stroke, myocardial infarction, or vascular death in a nondiabetic and diabetic study population (ADA – Aspirin Therapy 2004). Aspirin and clopidogrel are sometimes combined.

A recent systemic review found that relative risk of intracranial haemorrhage in patients treated with thrombolytic therapy was about 50% greater in Afro-Caribbean patients when compared to nonblack patients (McDowell et al 2006).

RECOMMENDATIONS

There is a clear consensus between the recommendations produced by JBS 2 (Wood et al 2005), the ADA (ADA 2007) and Diabetes UK that, unless contraindicated, aspirin should be prescribed in the dose range 75 to 150 mg to all patients with type 2 diabetes **and** existing CVD. Diabetes UK qualifies this with a lower age limit of 30 years (Diabetes UK 2001). Although all of these bodies recommend that, unless contraindicated, aspirin should be prescribed to most type 2 diabetics **without** evidence of CVD, the criteria vary:

For JBS 2, the criteria for prescribing a recommended dose of 75 mg are:

- All aged 50 years or more
- Under age 50 years with one of the following:
  - duration of disease more than 10 years
  - already receiving treatment for raised blood pressure
  - evidence of target organ damage (retinopathy and/or nephropathy) whose blood pressure is controlled to below 150/90.

For the ADA, the criteria for prescribing a recommended dose of 75 to 162 mg are:

- All aged over 40 years with the presence of an additional cardiovascular risk factor (such as family history of CVD, hypertension, smoking, dyslipidaemia and albuminuria).
- "Consider" aspirin therapy, unless contraindicated, in people aged 30 to 40 years with the presence of an additional cardiovascular risk factor.

For Diabetes UK, the criteria for prescribing a recommended dose of 75 mg are:

- All aged over 30 years with one or more additional cardiovascular risk factors, as above, but also a BMI greater than 25 kg/m^2 or more, South Asian ethnicity, or the presence of diabetic retinopathy.

In a 2006 clinical review, Marshall and Flyvberg go further than the above and recommend that low-dose "aspirin should be prescribed for patients aged over 40" (Marshall & Flyvberg 2006). Bearing in mind that type 2 diabetics require an approach based upon secondary prevention interventions (even in the absence of CVD) and that aspirin is under-prescribed, this recommendation has considerable merit.

In order to minimise the risk of the patient having a cerebro-vascular event, it is recommended that aspirin is started only when blood pressure is controlled to less than 150/90. Aspirin should not be prescribed to individuals under the age of 21 years, because of the increased risk of Reye's syndrome associated with aspirin use in young people.

OTHER RISK FACTORS

AGE

Cardiovascular disease risk and the prevalence of type 2 diabetes both increase with age: this may be due, in a large part, to the greater prevalence of adverse cardiovascular risk factors with increasing age. The increased incidence of CVD with age is incremental rather than linear. It is more worrying (but not surprising) that the onset of CVD occurs at a younger average age in the diabetic population.

GENDER

If the profile of other risk factors is otherwise similar, then healthy pre-menopausal females should be at less risk of developing CVD than their male contemporaries. However, in diabetic pre-menopausal females, this normally protective cardiovascular effect is lost (Barrett-Connor et al 1991). There is evidence that the presence of a cardiovascular risk factor sometimes has a greater adverse effect upon women than upon men when diabetes is present: for example, women appear to be more susceptible to the adverse effects of both active and passive smoking upon cardiovascular risk.

A meta-analysis of prospective cohort studies concluded that the excess risk for fatal CHD mortality associated with diabetes is greater in women (3.5 odds ratio) than in men (2.06 odds ratio) and the "adjusted pool" ratio of relative risks in women compared to men was 1.46. However, the analysis could not adjust for menopausal status (and hormone replace therapy) and duration of diabetes, which may be potential confounding factors (Huxley et al 2006).

The authors went on to postulate about the reasons for why this adverse effect was greater in women than in men:

- Women with diabetes not only had significantly higher blood pressure and lipid levels than men with diabetes, but also the differences among people with and without diabetes were greater in women than in men.
- Since men with diabetes or CVD are more likely to be taking aspirin, statins or antihypertensive drugs than women, there may be a treatment bias that favours men.

ETHNICITY

Due to complex and not entirely understood reasons, type 2 diabetes and CHD are commoner in certain ethnic groups, particularly in Indo-Asians, Afro-Caribbeans, Hispanic-Americans, Native Americans, Fijians and many other non-white populations. This increased prevalence appears to be due to a combination of greater prevalence of other cardiovascular risk factors (which also produces greater insulin resistance), and an increased vulnerability to the effects of these risk factors. However, the presence of diabetes increases the prevalence of underlying CVD in *all* populations, irrespective of the level of original risk.

Another aspect of ethnicity in respect to CVD that needs to borne in mind is that the risk of adverse reactions occurring to some cardiovascular drugs may vary between ethnic groups. Although sound clinical judgement must be the basis of any treatment decisions and considerably more research is needed, clinicians should be aware of potentially variable outcomes to drug treatment within the context of a risk assessment for that intervention (Eliasson 2006).

POSITIVE FAMILY HISTORY

Patients with a family history of premature arteriosclerosis are at greater risk of developing CVD, particularly in a first-degree relative, i.e. parent, sibling or child. This may be due largely to the increased prevalence (genetically mediated) of other adverse cardiovascular risk factors and an increased vulnerability to their effects. However, some families may also be exposed to one or more common adverse environmental components.

AN "ALTERNATIVE" VIEW OF TARGETS

Two papers (Winocour 2002, Law & Wald 2002), published in the same issue of the *British Medical Journal* in 2002, analysed the benefits and problems associated with striving to achieve the targets advised by the various expert bodies and performance contracts.

QOF ◄
DM7
DM12
DM17
DM20

Two problems of striving to reach a fixed target set for all patients, irrespective of their baseline prior to intervention, are:

1. The current targets set started as a mean and were achieved only by 50 to 70% of subjects in research studies.
2. Attaining these targets required polypharmacy, with the drawbacks of potentially reduced concordance and increased likelihood of drug interactions.

Given the typical cardiovascular risk profile of many type 2 diabetics and the tight recommended targets that need to be achieved, professionals could be prescribing simultaneously **eight** drugs:

- **two** hypoglycaemic agents
- **three** antihypertensive agents
- **two** lipid-modifying agents

    and

- **aspirin**

    in addition to prescribing for other medical problems!

Many patients would find such a regimen unacceptable or difficult. The factors that influence concordance are complex and vary between individual patients. Both once- and twice-daily regimens are associated with better concordance than three or more daily doses. Once-daily dosing has the advantage over twice-daily of reducing the tablet "load". However, in patients known to miss medication, twice-daily dosing may result in shorter periods of sub-therapeutic medication levels (Wright 1993). Medication regimens may be simplified by combining more than one active drug in a single agent. There is evidence to suggest that fixed-dose combination pills and unit-of-use packaging are likely to improve adherence, although this has not been quantified (Connor et al 2004). Providing patients with a pocket-sized tablet dispenser holding one day's tablets in up to three doses has been shown to improve adherence and glycaemic control (Maier et al 2006).

Winacour proposed alternative targets for glycaemic and blood pressure control (see Table 4.11). It may be preferable to set pragmatic individualised targets, in full collaboration with the patient and aiming to improve the adverse measurement of each component, rather than to pursue inflexibly several simultaneous "tough" targets.

Law and Wald argue that variables, such as blood pressure, serum cholesterol, and body mass index, have a dose–response relationship with the diseases that they "cause". They also argue "that a given change in the variables reduces the risk of disease by a constant proportion of the existing risk irrespective of the starting level of

TABLE 4.11 Targets for certain measurable components of diabetes care (Winocour & Fisher 2003)

Component	Current recommendations	Alternative recommendation: for an individual	Alternative recommendation: for the clinic
HbA1c	7.0–7.5%	a. 6.5% within 3 years of diagnosis, if no complications, on diet b. 8% 5 years after diagnosis, if complications c. 9% insulin treated obese	a. 50% <7.5% b. & c. reduction in clinic mean by 10–20%
Blood pressure	130–140/80–85	a. 160/95 if aged >75 b. 150/90 if CHD, microalbuminuria, dyslipidaemia or smoker c. Reduce BP by 10–20%	a. 140/90 in 40% of treated patients b. 160/95 in 75% of treated patients c. Shift clinic mean by 10–20%

the variable or existing risk", concluding that a patient's overall absolute level of risk, not the level of individual risk factors, should determine the threshold for intervention. If a patient is at high risk, then appropriate intervention targets should require substantial changes in all reversible risk factors simultaneously. This is supported by the findings from the MRC/BHF Heart Protection Study that high-risk patients benefited from statin treatment, irrespective of pre-treatment cholesterol levels (Collins et al 2002). Greater risk reduction results from a significant change that falls short of reaching a fixed endpoint than from minimal change that does reach that endpoint.

Whatever targets are set and whatever interventions are undertaken, it is important what is measured accurately reflects what is and should be done. It is easier, but not necessarily preferable, to collect data about whether fixed end points have been reached (usually one measurement) than to measure how much change has occurred (which requires an additional measurement and calculation). Robert McNamara, the American Secretary of Defense in the 1960s, advised to avoid, "making what is measurable important, and find ways of making the important measurable".

Perhaps, the important messages are that:

1. Targets should be set at a realistic and achievable level for the individual patient.
2. All treatable cardiovascular risk factors should be tackled in patients identified as "high risk".
3. Any improvement in a risk factor is likely to produce some benefit, whatever the starting point.

► KEY POINTS

- All patients with type 2 diabetes are at increased cardiovascular risk (when compared to the nondiabetic population).

- The most important modifiable cardiovascular risk factors are smoking, raised blood pressure, dyslipidaemia, increased waist circumference, physical inactivity and increased platelet adhesiveness.

- Treating all of these has been shown to reduce cardiovascular risk in diabetics.

- The greatest benefit will come from attacking aggressively all relevant risk factors, irrespective of the baseline, and not from an excessive focus on one factor to the possible exclusion of others.

- Pharmacotherapy for lowering blood pressure often requires combinations of drugs. The extent of lowering is probably more important than which drug(s) is (are) used.

- Lowering both total and LDL cholesterol with a statin is the mainstay of lipid modification, but other approaches may be required, particularly if the aim is to raise HDL cholesterol.

- Waist circumference is a better indicator of obesity than BMI. Anti-obesity drugs are often effective, but surgery is being increasingly used in the most extreme cases.

- Low-dose aspirin is indicated in many people with type 2 diabetes.

- The targets set for each risk factor need to be both realistic and individual for the patient.

DIABETES COMPLICATIONS

OVERVIEW

NSF
11
12

In this section, specific complications associated with diabetes are discussed. Most of the mechanisms are vascular and the interventions will include components that reduce cardiovascular risk or improve glycaemic control. The assessment and interventions should be structured and follow agreed pathways.

EYES

RATIONALE

QOF
DM

Diabetes has long been associated with eye problems, including retinopathy, cataracts and glaucoma. Individually or collectively, these problems can lead to visual loss. Diabetic retinopathy is a specific vascular complication of diabetes and is the most common cause of newly registered cases of blindness (12%) in those aged 20 to 64 years in the UK (Evans et al 1991). In type 2 diabetics, glaucoma and cataracts are a more frequent cause of visual loss than retinopathy, but the latter is already present at diagnosis in one-fifth of patients (Macleod et al 1994) and its prevalence relates directly to the duration of diabetes.

Among the risk factors associated with the development and progression of diabetic retinal disease in type 2 diabetics are: raised blood pressure (UKPDS 1998c), increased duration of diabetes (Klein et al 1984), and the presence of microalbuminuria (Savage et al 1996).

The St Vincent Declaration of 1989 set a target to reduce new blindness caused by diabetes by one-third or more (Krans et al 1995). Regular accurate screening for diabetic eye disease can improve the prognosis by detecting abnormalities earlier in their natural history. Active management of micro-angiopathy affecting the retina has been possible since the development of laser photocoagulation. Cataract surgery and other surgical techniques that may benefit patients with diabetic eye disease are now available.

TARGETS

The aims of a screening and management programme for diabetic eye disease should be to:

- Prevent or delay the onset of diabetic retinopathy
- Detect at the earliest opportunity any treatable abnormalities in the lens and/or retina by population-based, high-quality screening
- Treat effectively any diabetic eye disease present
- Preserve visual function.

SCREENING

Programmes

The two preferred methods of screening for diabetic retinopathy that meet the National Clinical Guidelines' recommendation of a sensitivity of at least 80% and a specificity of at least 95% (Hutchinson et al 2001) are:

1. A suitably trained assessor (optician, GP with ophthalmological experience), using mydriatic slit-lamp indirect ophthalmoscopy

   or

2. Mydriatic retinal photography (first choice), where the images are evaluated by trained retinal scorers (although there is still considerable regional variation in practice across the UK).

If a practice does not have access to either a slit-lamp or a retinal photography service, **only** suitably trained personnel should screen retinas using direct ophthalmoscopy (i.e. an ophthalmoscope) with mydriasis (pupil dilatation), although the reported sensitivity and specificity are lower for this method than the recommended minimum above and direct ophthalmoscopy risks missing clinically significant macular oedema (CSMO).

The National Screening Committee recommended that a diabetic retinopathy screening programme should:

- Undertake an annual programme for all those with diabetes
- Have an integral quality assurance framework
- Be integrated with the other local programmes for diabetes care.

The preferred screening methods are more likely to meet these criteria.

Retinopathy screening has been an early high priority in the Diabetes NSF: a stated aim was to offer it to 80% of diabetics by March 2006, rising to 100% by the end of 2007. At the time of writing, it is unclear how successful the NHS has been at meeting this aim. The data from the QOF reviews do not indicate which screening methods have been used.

Visual acuity

Assessing visual acuity has limited value in detecting diabetic retinopathy, since not all retinopathy affects vision, especially if the macula is spared. When done, the clinician should use a properly illuminated Snellen chart of correct size for 3 or 6 metres and a pinhole to correct refractory errors.

Fundoscopy

If undertaking direct ophthalmoscopy to screen for diabetic retinopathy, the following sequence should be followed:

1. Before dilating pupils with 1% tropicamide, first check:
   - the depth of the anterior chambers (shining a torch from the side at a right angle should illuminate the whole of the iris) to exclude any increased risk of provoking acute angle closure
   - that the patient is aware that he or she should not drive for approximately 6 hours after the drops (although there is debate about the extent to which mydriasis can affect driving vision)
2. Allow at least 10 minutes for drops to work, after which check red reflex
3. Start with holding the ophthalmoscope 50 cm in front of each eye, and adjust the focus to look for corneal scars, lens opacities and vitreous haemorrhage
4. Slowly move closer to the patient in order to examine the retina systematically:
   - start at the optic disc, looking for new vessels or cupping (evidence of glaucoma)
   - locate the macula and check the surrounding area for haemorrhages and exudates (especially hard exudates in a circular pattern)
   - follow the major veins from the optic disc out to the periphery looking for venous irregularities (e.g. beading) and new vessels
   - inspect elsewhere in the retina for haemorrhages, exudates, fibrous tissue or detachment.

The findings of the examination will determine the classification of diabetic retinopathy, as outlined in Figure 5.1.

INTERVENTIONS

The appropriate management of diabetic retinopathy should follow the pathway outlined in Table 5.1.

Suitable interventions that can be undertaken in primary care include:

- *Modification of risk factors* (tighter glycaemic and blood pressure control). It is advisable to stabilise sight-threatening retinal disease first, as rapid improvement in glycaemic control can result in the short-term worsening of diabetic retinal disease. However, tight blood glucose control has been shown to reduce the progression of diabetic retinopathy (requiring retinal photocoagulation) and the deterioration of visual acuity in type 2 diabetics (Stratton et al 2000). Aspirin use, in the absence of contraindications, should be considered.
- *Appropriate referral to secondary care*, depending upon the degree of retinopathy found or whether cataracts interfere with vision.
- *Rehabilitation* may involve community support, low-vision aids and training in their use for patients with visual impairment.

Secondary-care interventions may include the following:

- *Laser photocoagulation* for high-risk retinopathy (moderately proliferative or worse) and CSMO (focal or modified grid laser)
- *Vitrectomy* may be considered in type 2 diabetics who have a vitreous haemorrhage too severe to allow laser photocoagulation

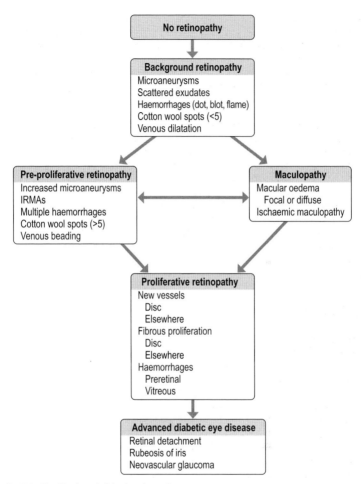

Fig. 5.1 Classification of diabetic retinopathy

- *Cataract extraction*, the outcome of which is closely linked to age and severity of retinopathy present before surgery
- *Intravitreal steroids*, which is not without risks
- A potential new treatment is *Ruboxistaurin*, an oral protein kinase C inhibitor, which is showing promise in trials in patients with CSMO.

TABLE 5.1 Management pathways following eye assessment (NICE 2002a, UK National Screening Committee 2004)

Care pathway	Visual acuity	Lens	Retina*	Other factors
Routine review (1 year)	Unchanged	Clear or minimal opacities	No changes or minimal/low-risk background	
Early review (3–6 months)			New or worsening lesions or exudates >1 dd from fovea	Renal disease or rapid improvement of blood glucose
Routine referral to ophthalmologist		Cataracts interfering with vision	View is obscured (but beware of possibility of significant retinopathy)	
Sooner referral (within 12 weeks) to ophthalmologist	Unexplained drop		Hard exudates <1 dd from fovea or macular oedema or unexplained findings or pre-proliferative retinopathy or more advanced (severe) retinopathy	
Urgent referral (within 2 weeks) to ophthalmologist			New vessels	Pre-retinal and/or vitreous haemorrhage Rubeosis iridis
Emergency referral (same day) to ophthalmologist	Sudden loss		Retinal detachment	

*dd, disc diameter

NEPHROPATHY

RATIONALE

Diabetic nephropathy is one of the more serious complications of diabetes. It occurs in 20–40% of patients with diabetes and its prevalence is increasing. Indo-Asian and Afro-Caribbean type 2 diabetics are at a greater risk of developing diabetic nephropathy than whites. In England, the rates for initiating treatment for end-stage renal disease were reported as 4.2 and 3.7 times higher in Afro-Caribbeans and Indo-Asians, respectively, than in whites (Roderick et al 1996).

Persistent albumin excretion greater than 300 mg/day, termed *macroalbuminuria*, in the absence of infection, marks the onset of diabetic nephropathy, and is also associated with increased mortality, particularly from vascular causes (Macleod et al 1995). The natural history of overt diabetic nephropathy is to progress to end-stage renal failure. The presence of lesser amounts of urinary albumin (less than 300 mg/day), termed *microalbuminuria*, indicates early renal damage. This is a risk factor for cardiovascular morbidity and mortality in type 2 diabetics (Dinneen & Gerstein 1997). About half of diabetics develop microalbuminuria at some stage. Of these (the study's subjects were on insulin) 30–50% will progress to macroalbuminuria, but 30–50% will revert to normal albumin excretion and 20–30% will continue to have microalbuminuria (Laing et al 2003). If retinopathy is also present, then diabetes-related renal disease is the likely cause of the albuminuria. If retinopathy is absent, other causes of renal disease should be considered (NICE 2002b).

Prompt and effective interventions, particularly at an early stage, may both prevent end-stage renal failure and reduce the high risk of cardiovascular disease. The management of chronic kidney disease is now the subject of an NSF published in 2005 (DH Renal NSF Team 2006).

AIM

The overriding aim is to identify and manage patients at increased risk of premature vascular disease and of diabetic nephropathy, and to reduce their risk of progressing to end-stage renal failure.

SCREENING

Screening for diabetic nephropathy should check at least annually two parameters:

1. Urinary albumin excretion
2. Estimated glomerular filtration rate (eGFR) or serum creatinine from a blood sample.

Urinary albumin (including microalbuminuria)

The categorisation of levels of albumin excretion is explained in Table 5.2.

TABLE 5.2 Levels of urinary albumin excretion	
Category	Spot collection (ng/ml creatinine)
Normal	<30
Microalbuminuria	30–299
Macro- (clinical) albuminuria	300 or more

The "gold standard" for the measurement of urinary albumin excretion is a timed urine sample (either over 24 hours, enabling simultaneous measurement of creatinine clearance, or 4 hours), but this is not a practical screening procedure for widespread use in the community.

Sending an early morning urine sample (also referred to as a "spot check") to a chemical pathology laboratory to measure the albumin:creatinine ratio (ACR) is both more practical and the preferred method recommended by the ADA. ACR levels equal to or greater than 2.5 mg/mmol in males or 3.5 mg/mmol in females indicate microalbuminuria. The test needs to be repeated for confirmation, as microalbuminuria can be transient. One of the authors completed a study in which the prevalence of microalbuminuria in diabetics in an ethnically mixed UK community was 19.3%. The characteristics independently associated with a higher prevalence of microalbuminuria were current insulin use, current smoking, older age, higher systolic blood pressure and poorer metabolic control, but there was no significant association with either increasing duration or gender. Unfortunately, the sample size was not large enough to determine whether there was an association between microalbuminuria and Indo-Asian ethnicity (Levene et al 2004).

Estimated glomerular filtration rate

From 2006 the reporting of estimated glomerular filtration rate (eGFR) has replaced the measurement of serum creatinine as standard in most laboratories. This change follows the recommendation of the Renal NSF. Serum creatinine levels may be affected by several factors, including age, gender, ethnicity, muscle mass, diet and some medications. Although not perfect, the eGFR is believed to be a better measure of renal function and easier for patients to understand than a serum creatinine result.

The glomerular filtration rate can be calculated using a formula and has been proposed as a more accurate, but logistically feasible, estimation of renal function. The 4-variable Modification of Diet and Renal Disease (MDRD) (Levey et al 1999) formula uses the patient's creatinine, age (valid only between 18 and 70 years), sex and race:

GFR (ml/min/1.73 m^2) = 175 × (S$_{cr}$/88.4)$^{-1.154}$ × (age)$^{-0.203}$ × (0.742 if female) × (1.210 if black), where S$_{cr}$ is the plasma creatinine expressed in μmol/l (SI units)

Pathology laboratories have started reporting eGFR automatically (with white ethnicity as default) using the MDRD formula: the result must be multiplied by 1.21 if the patient is black African. If the laboratory does not provide an eGFR result or if looking at a historical creatinine result, then eGFR can be calculated using a readily available online calculator: http://www.kidney.org/professionals/kdoqi/gfr_calculator.cfm.

Since glomerular filtration rate is affected by the body's surface area and the eGFR's calculation does not include this, an eGFR result can underestimate renal function in large people and underestimate it in slim small people.

The Renal NSF classifies those with kidney disease into 5 stages, based upon eGFR and the presence of urinary albumin (see Table 5.3).

TABLE 5.3 Classification into CKD stages 1 to 5, based upon estimated glomerular filtration ratio (eGFR)

Stage	eGFR (ml/min)	Other
1	≥90	Haematuria or proteinuria must be present
2	60–89	Haematuria or proteinuria must be present
3	30–59	
4	15–29	
5	≤15 or renal replacement therapy	

MANAGEMENT

A number of interventions have been shown to delay the progression of diabetic nephropathy.

Management can be divided into nonpharmacological and pharmacological:

Nonpharmacological
Smoking cessation
This also reduces CVD risk.

Optimising glycaemic control
The UKPDS found that intensive diabetes management with the goal of achieving near normoglycemia delayed the onset of microalbuminuria and the progression of micro- to macro-albuminuria in type 2 diabetics (UKPDS 1998a, b).

Dietary protein restriction
There are "no RCTs evaluating the effects of protein restriction in people with type 2 diabetes and … nephropathy on the outcomes of all cause mortality, incidence of end stage renal disease, or incidence of cardiovascular events" (Clinical Evidence online).

Pharmacological
Lowering blood pressure
Tight blood pressure control is the most important intervention for delaying the development of diabetic nephropathy (UKPDS 1998c). The target is a diastolic blood pressure below 75 mmHg in "normotensive insulin-dependent" or 90 mmHg in "hypertensive non-insulin-dependent" (BNF).

There is strong evidence for the reno-protective effect of ACE inhibitors/ARBs which have a greater effect upon urinary albumin excretion, a stronger marker for renal disease and cardiovascular health, than other blood-pressure-lowering drug classes. A Cochrane review suggests that ACE inhibitors are the best drug class to prevent microalbuminuria and nephropathy (Strippoli et al 2005). One randomised controlled trial (RCT), whose subjects were people with type 2 diabetes, hypertension, and microalbuminuria, reported that, compared with placebo, an ARB (irbesartan) reduced progression from early to late nephropathy over 2 years (Parving et al 2001). Another RCT, whose subjects were people with type 2 diabetes and early nephropathy found no significant difference in glomerular filtration rate change, mortality, or cardiovascular disease (CVD) events between an ARB (telmisartan) and an ACE inhibitor (enalapril) over 5 years (Barnett et al 2004). Other studies have found ARBs to be reno-protective in patients with type 2 diabetes and overt nephropathy (Brenner et al 2001, Lewis et al 2001).

However, effective blood pressure control is paramount, and non-DCCBs, β-blockers, or diuretics should be used in combination with or, if ACE inhibitor/ARB is contraindicated or not tolerated, as alternatives to inhibition of the renin-angiotensin-aldosterone system (Black et al 2003, Pepine et al 2003).

Low-dose aspirin
Unless contraindicated, low-dose aspirin (75 mg per day) should be taken by patients with diabetic nephropathy to reduce cardiovascular risk.

Improving lipid profile
Prescribing a statin reduces cardiovascular risk in patients with diabetic nephropathy.

The small Danish Steno-2 study compared the effect of a targeted, intensified, multifactorial (both lifestyle and pharmacological) intervention with that of conventional treatment on modifiable risk factors for CVD in type 2 diabetics and microalbuminuria, showing significantly reduced hazard ratios for the development of both macro- and microvascular complications in type 2 diabetics with microalbuminuria (Gaede et al 2003).

Monitoring serum potassium
Abnormal potassium levels can occur for a variety of reasons in patients with diabetes, and with or without nephropathy. **Hyperkalaemia** (serum potassium above the upper reference limit, usually 5.5 mEq/l) can result from ACE inhibitors, ARBs or potassium-sparing diuretics, and may occur in renal impairment. **Hypokalaemia** (serum potassium below the lower reference limit, usually 3.5 mEq/l) can result from long-term thiazide treatment without potassium-sparing medication or supplement. Treatment aims to restore normokalaemia.

Referral
If renal function deteriorates in patients with diabetic nephropathy (particularly to CKD Stages 4 or 5), then referral to a specialist nephropathy team may be appropriate for the following reasons:

1. Optimising medical management
2. Determining if a component of renovascular disease is present. Angioplasty to improve renal perfusion may preserve renal function
3. Preparing patients for dialysis (usually chronic ambulatory peritoneal dialysis), which is increasing performed in diabetics.

Patients with CKD stage 3 may need referral, depending on the presence of other morbidities or failure to respond to the interventions described above.

FEET

See also the subsection on neuropathy.

QOF ◄
DM9
DM10

RATIONALE

Definition

WHO has defined the diabetic foot as a group of syndromes in which neuropathy, ischaemia and infection lead to tissue breakdown, resulting in morbidity and possible amputation (Krans et al 1995).

Pathological processes

Peripheral neuropathy causes lost sensation and autonomic dysfunction. Peripheral vascular disease (atherosclerosis of large and/or small leg vessels) causes ischaemia. Trauma (which may involve altered pressure-loading and be unnoticed by the patient) followed by infection complicates neuropathy and ischaemia to cause significant tissue damage, such as ulceration.

There are two main pathological pathways in diabetic feet:

- *Neuropathic feet* have good circulation (pulses are present) and are warm, dry, numb and usually painless. The two main complications are neuropathic ulcers (commonly on the soles) and neuropathic (Charcot) joints. Rapidly spreading infection can result in massive tissue destruction, the main indication for amputation in neuropathic feet.
- *Neuro-ischaemic feet* are also numb, but cool, and the pulses are absent. In addition to the above neuropathic complications, pain at rest, ulcers at the edges, which result from trauma such as pressure damage, and gangrene may occur.

In both groups, the sequence of minor trauma, cutaneous ulceration and finally failure of the wound to heal can eventually lead to amputation, particularly if infection sets in, and rapid and significant tissue destruction occurs.

In diabetics attending dedicated foot clinics, approximately 50% have neuropathic feet and 50% have neuro-ischaemic feet (Edmonds et al 1986).

The burden of diabetic foot problems

A UK population-based study in type 2 patients gave a prevalence of 1.4% for foot ulcers, but the prevalence of the risk factors that give rise to ulcers was 41.6% (Kumar et al 1994). Once a limb has been amputated the prognosis for the contralateral limb is poor (Ebskov & Josephsen 1980). Foot ulcers occur more frequently in whites than in Indo-Asians or Afro-Caribbeans, and are associated with adverse social circumstances such as deprivation and isolation (Boulton 1997), poor glycaemic control, the presence of other vascular risk factors (e.g. smoking) and increased duration of diabetes.

Up to 50% of foot ulcers and amputations could be prevented by patient education and effective intervention (Boulton 1997). Diabetes complications consume considerable resource (both health and social costs). There are no current UK estimates for the costs of treating diabetic foot problems.

AIMS

Diabetic foot care must seek to prevent foot ulcers and gangrene (leading to amputation). However, this aim can be subdivided into:

1. Provision of suitable health education that increases the patient's ability to self-manage effectively with prompt appropriate illness-seeking behaviour in the presence of suspected pathology.
2. Identifying patients who have either a high risk (presence of neuropathy and/or peripheral vascular disease) of developing, or the presence of, lower-limb complications (e.g. foot ulcer, gangrene).
3. Optimal management of these patients to minimise morbidity, especially amputation.

ASSESSMENT

Assessment should be undertaken regularly by suitably trained professionals. The assessment process needs to be systematic with the aim of identifying the level of risk to the foot and, thus, ensuring that the appropriate management can be undertaken to prevent or minimise complications. Information gathering involves both a history and an examination.

History

The professional should also look for factors that may affect the patient's ability to self-manage. The following may be useful to elicit:

- Any *sensory symptoms*, such as pain, numbness, coldness, or tingling
- Any *associated physical problems*, such as poor visual acuity or mobility that can adversely affect self care
- *Concurrent diabetes complications* (nephropathy, retinopathy – hopefully apparent from the rest of the review or medical records) *and risk factors* (smoking, alcohol)

- A *previous history of increased or high-risk diabetic foot* (such as infection or foot ulcer), which may be documented in the medical records
- The patient's *understanding* of preventive foot care
- The patient's *social circumstances*.

Examination

The four main components of a routine structured foot examination of a person with diabetes are:

1. Testing of foot sensation.
   Neuropathy can be identified either by testing sensation threshold using a 10 g monofilament (light, easy to use and cheap – use on 10 patients before allowing 24 hours for filament to recover) **or** by testing vibration threshold using either a calibrated tuning fork or a biothesiometer (requires a power source and costs about £400).
2. Palpation of foot pulses
   However, it should be remembered that pulse assessment in an oedematous, ulcerated foot may be impossible, and infection of foot ulcers due to neuropathy often masks the subtle signs of arterial insufficiency, e.g. skin colour changes associated with elevation or lowering of the foot. Measuring the ankle-brachial pressure ratio (ABPR) in diabetics with Doppler may be misleading, due to calcification: it should be undertaken only in specialist clinics
3. Inspection of any foot deformity
4. Inspection of footwear (McIntosh et al 2003).

More details of each of these examination components are given in Table 5.4.

A range of risk factors are associated with the development of diabetic foot disease or ulcers. These include:

- Peripheral vascular disease (including previous vascular surgery)
- Neuropathy
- Foot deformities
- Plantar callus
- Visual impairment
- Smoking
- Physical disability (e.g. cardiovascular accident, gross obesity).

Ideally, the examination will correctly identify:

- The presence of neuropathy, circulatory impairment or abnormal pressure that puts the foot "at risk"
- A serious diabetic foot problem, such as ulcer, infection (cellulitis, abscess and/or osteomyelitis) or gangrene.

Critical ischaemia is characterised by rest or night pain *or* pale/mottled foot *or* dependent rubor *or* ischaemic ulceration *or* gangrene. *Severe infection* is characterised by the presence of abscess *or* cellulitis.

TABLE 5.4 Examination of the diabetic foot

Inspect footwear for suitability and for evidence of excessive wear or pressure loading. Inspect distal lower limbs, looking for:

- Foot deformity, callus formation at pressure areas (increased risk of trauma)
- Distended foot veins (associated with autonomic neuropathy)
- Small muscle wasting (associated with somatic neuropathy)
- Oedema (associated with impaired circulation)
- Hair loss (associated with impaired circulation)
- Colour changes (pallor associated with ischaemia; erythema associated with cellulitis)
- Ulcerative lesions (neuropathic more likely on the sole; ischaemic more likely on the toe tips and/or dorsum)
- Other serious lesions, such as abscess, osteomyelitis or gangrene

Check for evidence of neuropathy:

- Decreased vibration sensation using a 128 Hz tuning fork, or a biothesiometer (if available)
- Decreased skin pressure perception threshold using a 10 g (5.07) monofilament, which is pushed perpendicularly against the skin on the sole of the foot until it buckles; inability to feel the filament applied in this way indicates a greater risk of developing a foot ulcer (McIntosh et al 2003)
- Decreased ankle reflexes
- Dry and warm skin may indicate autonomic neuropathy

Check for evidence of impaired circulation:

- Reduced or absent pulses: in proximal disease femoral pulses are weak and more distal pulses are absent; in distal disease, which occurs more often in diabetics, femoral and popliteal pulses are normal, but foot pulses are absent
- Decreased skin temperature
- Foot whitens when held elevated for 30 seconds
- If available, Doppler can be used to quantify the extent of arterial obstruction by measuring blood pressure in the lower limb

Check for evidence of musculoskeletal abnormalities:

- Is the range of movement of ankle joint and foot normal?
- Analysis of gait and stance abnormalities may suggest trauma and/or tissue damage

---

Charcot osteoarthropathy

Charcot osteoarthropathy is a progressive condition, associated with neuropathy in diabetics. It is characterised by dislocation of joints, fractures and destruction of the bony architecture. In diabetics, the arch of the foot is most frequently affected. Trauma (even through simple weight bearing) in a severely neuropathic limb is thought to trigger Charcot's osteoarthropathy. Although not particularly common, it is a major risk factor for foot ulceration and amputation. If suspected, the patient should be referred promptly to the multidisciplinary foot care management team, where the management includes immobilisation of the affected joint and long-term off-loading to prevent ulceration (McIntosh et al 2003).

Categorisation of level of risk

Based upon the information acquired from the history and examination, the level of current risk to the diabetic foot of developing a foot disease or ulcer can be determined. NICE in 2003 has defined the features and management at each level of risk (McIntosh et al 2003). A fifth level (number 5) is added to this categorisation.

The levels of risk are:

1. In a foot at **low risk**, all of the following are present: normal sensation, palpable pulses, no deformity, no skin lesions. Also there is no previous history of diabetic foot ulcer.
2. In a foot at **increased risk**, *one* of the following is present: neuropathy or absent pulses (or previous vascular surgery) or a risk factor.
3. In a foot at **high risk**, neuropathy or absent pulses *plus* skin changes or deformity or previous ulcer (caused by neuropathy and/or ischaemia) are present. A history of previous amputation can also be considered as an indicator of a high-risk foot.
4. In a foot with **active disease**, either an active foot ulcer or difficult to control painful neuropathy or a Charcot osteoarthropathy is present.
5. An **emergency foot problem** is when either critical ischaemia or severe infection is present.

The severity of a foot ulcer is classified according to the Wagner system, summarised in Table 5.5 (Wagner 1983).

MANAGEMENT

The level of risk to the diabetic foot determines the optimal management pathway, summarised in Table 5.6.

TABLE 5.5 Wagner classification of foot ulceration (Wagner 1983)	
Grade	Description
0	High-risk foot; no ulcers
1	Superficial ulcer (skin deep), not clinically infected
2	Deeper ulcer, often with cellulitis; no abscess or bony involvement
3	Deep ulcer with abscess or bony involvement (osteomyelitis)
4	Localised gangrene (involving toe, forefoot or heel)
5	Gangrene of the entire foot

TABLE 5.6 Summary of management pathways for diabetic feet (modified from McIntosh 2003 foot care guidelines)

Level of risk	Management
Low risk	Agree management plan, including foot-care education Trained patient undertakes own nail care Arrange recall and annual review as part of ongoing care
Increased risk	Surveillance by podiatrist or practice nurse with increased training Recall and review every 3 to 6 months
High risk	Refer to podiatrist with special interest in diabetes *or* to local hospital-based specialist diabetes team Recall and review every 1 to 3 months
Active foot disease	Refer urgently to multidisciplinary foot-care team (within 24 hours)
Emergency foot problem	Admission for in-patient care

Management options in primary care

Even when the patient is under active specialist care, there are a number of appropriate interventions that can and should be undertaken in a primary care setting.

Health education

This is an essential component and needs to be on-going, whatever the level of risk. Table 5.7 lists the important health education messages concerning foot care that need to be delivered to diabetics. This can be given by the GP or practice nurse (if suitably trained) or by the podiatrist.

Optimising glycaemic control

Poor glycaemic control is associated with a greater risk of microvascular complications (UKPDS 1998b).

Improved management of other cardiovascular risk factors

The interventions may include low-dose aspirin, lowering blood pressure, encouraging smoking cessation, and improving the lipid profile. Patients with peripheral vascular disease probably have widespread atheroma and, therefore, are also at a higher risk of developing cardiovascular disease.

Debridement

Patients with neuropathic ulcers require frequent removal of any dead skin or callus, unless revascularisation is required. This should be carried out only by a suitably qualified podiatrist. There should be a very low threshold here for referral to secondary care, since "ordinary" podiatrists who are unfamiliar with diabetes care often do not debride ulcers effectively enough.

TABLE 5.7 Health education guidelines for foot care in diabetics (Leicestershire Health 1996)

Hygiene

Good hygiene is essential:
  at least twice-weekly bathing and gentle dryings
  socks or stockings should be changed daily, the foot inspected carefully for infection
  talc avoided

How to avoid problems

Do not wear constricting footwear
Do not walk bare foot, sit by an open fire or use hot water bottles
Do not wear garters; these can reduce blood supply to the feet
Do not self-treat corns or callosities; go to a state-registered podiatrist
Cut nails straight across and not too short
Do not cut toenails yourself if you have difficulty in managing
Examine feet regularly for possible injuries, using a mirror to inspect the soles
Shoes should be inspected before and after putting them on; ensure no grit or other objects are in the shoe; avoid wear of lining, insoles and heels
Proper fitting and selection are essential when buying new shoes:
  measure feet when standing; uppers should be of soft leather
  ensure enough room across the ball of the foot and around the toes to enable wiggling
  there should be some sort of fastening mechanism; soles should be of rubber or microcellular type
  avoid excessively high heels
  high-quality cushioned-sole trainers reduce plantar pressure more than ordinary shoes, but less than custom-built shoes
Keep feet warm in winter: natural fibre cotton and/or wool hosiery is better than nylon
Seek advice from podiatrist or doctor if you notice:
  any foot injuries
  any swelling or throbbing pain in any part of feet
  any colour changes in any part of feet
  any discharge of coloured fluid from your feet, especially from corns, calluses or beneath toenails
  undue numbness or prickling sensation in feet

Analgesia

Neuropathic pain often does not respond to conventional analgesia. Tricyclic antidepressants, the anticonvulsant carbamazepine, and topical capsaicin can be effective in reducing pain. Gabapentin and pregabalin are anticonvulsants that increasingly are being used successfully by pain management experts.

Antibiotics

Patients with foot infections require prompt and aggressive treatment with one or more broad-spectrum antibiotics. Ideally, the choice of antibiotic should be guided by culture and sensitivity results (where available) and response to treatment. Unfortunately, surface swabs have been shown to be unreliable for determining the nature of infection and the more reliable method of tissue biopsy is not available in primary care (O'Meara et al 2006).

A longer duration and higher dose of antibiotic is usually required because of the poorer tissue perfusion and delayed healing that occurs in diabetics. NICE found insufficient data to support recommending any particular antibiotic regimen (McIntosh et al 1993).

Rational prescribing
In patients with peripheral vascular disease, certain drug classes may be less safe, such as β-blockers and ACE/ARB (increased risk of renal artery stenosis).

Earlier review
Depending upon the nature of the problem, recall for an earlier review is indicated to prevent progression.

Referral
High-risk patients, with an active foot disease or with an emergency diabetic foot require a timely and appropriate referral to secondary care to reduce the risk of progression to a higher-level lesion and, ultimately and tragically, amputation.

Secondary care interventions
In addition to the above, the following interventions are available in secondary care:

Orthotics
Custom-built footwear or orthotic insoles should be used to reduce plantar callus thickness and the incidence of foot ulcer relapse in high-risk diabetic feet.

Dressings and topical agents
When a foot ulcer is **not** infected, protective bandaging may be appropriate. A good dressing needs to be effective within the closed environment of footwear without causing problems, such as plugging the wound, failing due to pressures of walking, preventing ulcer inspection and occupying too much space. A variety of dressings are available: NICE recommends that the choice should "match clinical experience, patient preference, and the site of the wound", with consideration of costs (McIntosh et al 1993).

Intravenous antibiotics
These are indicated in severe cellulitis.

Vascular surgery
Patients with tissue loss and arterial disease should be considered for arterial reconstruction or angioplasty by a vascular surgeon. These are more likely to succeed if proximal disease is present rather than the more common distal disease.

Off-loading

Redistribution of weight, using casts, is also known as off-loading. It may be used to protect the vulnerable foot, such as in Charcot's osteoarthropathy, unless there is severe ischaemia.

Other treatments

NICE's most recent footcare guidelines cited a current lack of trial evidence for **not** recommending the use of other available interventions in treatment of foot ulcers.

Following a patient's discharge from hospital, the GP and/or practice nurse should monitor closely these patients and continue to undertake the above-stated primary care interventions.

NEUROPATHY

RATIONALE

QOF ◀
DM10

It is thought that 30–50% of diabetics will develop chronic peripheral neuropathy over their lifetime, with 10–20% having severe symptoms (Tesfaye & Kempler 2005). Diabetic neuropathy is not a single homogeneous condition: its clinical manifestations are diverse. These can be either focal or diffuse, and can cause considerable morbidity and may contribute to premature mortality. The two most frequent presentations are:

1. Distal symmetric polyneuropathy (DPN)

   and

2. Autonomic neuropathy.

Neuropathies result from microangiopathy of the vasa nervorum. The development of diabetic neuropathy starts with *intraneural biochemical abnormalities*, which lead to *decreased nerve conduction velocity*, then to *clinical neuropathy* and end with *end-stage complications* caused by major irreversible derangements of the nerve structure and function. Autonomic neuropathy can affect every organ system in the body. Often the pathogenic process does not progress through all of the stages, and only the latter two stages are clinically apparent.

The early recognition and appropriate management of diabetic neuropathies may be important for the following reasons:

- Up to 50% of patients with distal symmetric polyneuropathy may be asymptomatic: therefore, at increased risk of inadvertent injury to insensate feet.
- Cardiovascular autonomic neuropathy does cause substantial morbidity and mortality.
- Treatable non-diabetic neuropathies may be present.

- There are several interventions available for symptomatic relief of DPN and autonomic neuropathy (see below).

AIMS

The aims of screening and prompt appropriate interventions are to prevent or delay the onset of further neuropathy, and to alleviate symptoms (e.g. pain), and to reduce the risk of sudden death or disability from cardiac autonomic neuropathy.

SCREENING

The diagnosis of diabetic neuropathy is mainly clinical. More details of the features of the various manifestations of diabetic neuropathy can be found in Table 5.8. Before attributing the neuropathy found to diabetes, nondiabetic causes of neuropathy should be considered, including uraemia, deficiencies (B12), alcohol, neoplasia, paraproteinaemia, Guillain-Barré syndrome and drugs such as nitrofurantoin. Nausea, vomiting and diarrhoea can be caused by infection.

History

The history should elicit the presence of neuropathic symptoms, such as pain, weakness, sensory dysfunction. There may be features that suggest a nondiabetic cause. The symptoms of autonomic dysfunction may be elicited during a review of systems, involving the skin, pupils, heart, or gastrointestinal and genitourinary systems.

A potentially worrying symptom of autonomic neuropathy can be loss of the warning symptoms of impending hypoglycaemia.

Examination

The extent and type of examination is likely to be dictated by the history. If autonomic neuropathy is present, then distal symmetric polyneuropathy is also likely to be present.

For the assessment of distal symmetric polyneuropathy, a variety of tests can be used, such as pinprick sensation, temperature and vibration perception (using a 128-Hz tuning fork), 10-g monofilament pressure sensation at the dorsal surface of both great toes (just proximal to the nail bed), and ankle jerks (decrease or absence). If both loss of 10-g monofilament perception and reduced vibration perception are found, then a foot ulcer is more likely to develop. Although a minimum of one clinical test is used for screening, the use of two tests will lead to a more accurate diagnosis. To assess focal and multi-focal neuropathy, the clinical examination needs to be done in areas indicated by the neurological symptoms.

A decreased heart rate in response to the Valsalva manoeuvre and/or an unchanged heart rate variation during deep breathing is evidence of autonomic neuropathy. Erratic glycaemic control can be associated with gastroparesis. Cardiac autonomic neuropathy may be suggested by resting tachycardia (greater than 100 beats per minute), orthostatic hypotension (a fall in systolic blood pressure greater than 20 mmHg upon standing), or other disturbances in autonomic nervous system function.

TABLE 5.8 Classification and features of diabetic neuropathies (modified from Macleod 1997)

Type of neuropathy	Features include
Distal symmetric polyneuropathy or *peripheral sensorimotor*	(Acute or chronic) symmetrical; mainly sensory Pain is sharp, stabbing or burning Paraesthesia of soles or hyperaesthesia Often has a stocking-glove distribution
Autonomic:	
Orthostasis	Dizziness; drop of >20 mmHg systolic BP when standing
Resting tachycardia	Pulse >100 beats/min at rest
Gustatory sweating	Abnormal facial sweating while eating
Gastroparesis	Nausea and vomiting
Change in bowel frequency	Diarrhoea (often nocturnal) or constipation
Bladder dysfunction	Recurrent UTI, incontinence, palpable bladder
Erectile dysfunction (see below also)	Loss of penile erection and/or retrograde ejaculation
Mononeuropathy:	Median carpal tunnel syndrome Cranial nerves (III, IV, VI, VII)
External nerve pressure	Radial, ulnar and peroneal nerve palsies associated with pain
Proximal motor	Severe pain, associated with poor control Paraesthesiae in the proximal lower limbs Muscle wasting

Investigations

Specialised investigations are sometimes indicated. Structural abnormalities in the gastro-intestinal tract may need to be excluded by either endoscopy or barium studies.

MANAGEMENT

The optimal management of diabetic neuropathy depends to some extent upon its type and presentation. Care should be taken to monitor any side effects of any medication used. Some neuropathies, such as cranial nerve mononeuropathy, can improve spontaneously within weeks to months.

The interventions available in primary care include:

Optimising glycaemic control

Maintaining optimal glycaemic control will not reverse neuropathy, but observational studies suggest that it may improve or delay worsening of neuropathy. It is also suggested that avoiding extreme blood glucose fluctuations may be helpful (ADA 2007).

Analgesia

Mild-to-moderate pain may respond to paracetamol or a nonsteroidal anti-inflammatory drug (if not contraindicated). However, more severe neuropathic pain may not respond to conventional analgesia.

Tricyclic antidepressants have been historically the drugs of choice (e.g. amitriptyline and nortriptyline) for neuropathic pain. Both a Cochrane systematic review (Saarto & Wiffen 2005) and a recent meta-analysis (Wong 2007) found these drugs to be effective for a variety of neuropathic pains, with best evidence for amitriptyline, but tricyclic antidepressants are not currently licensed for the treatment of diabetic neuropathy in either the UK or USA. Proximal motor neuropathic pain may be relieved by amitriptyline. Tricyclics are generally inexpensive, but their use may be limited by their side effects; they may also exacerbate some autonomic symptoms such as gastroparesis. The 5-hydroxytryptamine and norepinephrine reuptake inhibitor duloxetine has a license for the treatment of diabetic peripheral neuropathic pain. There is limited evidence for the effectiveness of selective serotonin reuptake inhibitor antidepressant drugs (SSRIs). Further studies are needed to identify the most effective antidepressant.

The antiepileptic drug *gabapentin* is licensed for the treatment of neuropathic pain, and is being used as an alternative to a tricyclic antidepressant, particularly by those with an interest in pain management. Gabapentin should be started at low dose, then titrated over days to weeks to a dosage that is well tolerated and produces symptomatic relief (one regimen is 300 mg day one, 300 mg twice daily day 2, then 300 mg three times daily, with increases of 300 mg subsequently, as necessary). *Pregabalin* is structurally related to gabapentin, but is longer acting and has recently been confirmed to be useful in painful diabetic neuropathy in a randomised controlled trial. It too is licensed for the treatment of neuropathic pain. The antiepileptic drugs *carbamazepine* and *phenytoin* are unlicensed, but may be useful for the relief of shooting or stabbing pain: however, adverse effects (including nausea and vomiting, dizziness, headache and confusion) can occur frequently with these drugs.

Topical capsaicin cream (0.075%) is licensed for painful diabetic neuropathy and may bring some relief, but its use may be limited by the intense burning sensation it can produce when first used. A systematic review found that capsaicin "has poor to moderate efficacy in the treatment of chronic neuropathic … pain. However, it may be useful in people who are unresponsive to, or intolerant of other treatments" (Mason et al 2004).

In intermediate-term studies neuropathic pain has been shown to respond better to opioid analgesics, such as *tramadol* and *oxycodone*, than to placebo (Eisenberg et al 2006). These have a role when other treatments have failed, but more research is needed to determine their long-term efficacy and safety.

Acupuncture

If available, this may be useful in treating diabetic neuropathy.

Psychological support

This is important, especially when the neuropathy is disabling.

Rehabilitation and education

This may be helpful, particularly when there is motor impairment.

Treatment of any non-diabetic causes

Appropriate treatment may reduce the symptoms and/or progression of the neuropathy.

Diabetic autonomic neuropathy

The wide variety of agents is used to relieve the symptoms of autonomic neuropathy, which include:

- The mineralocorticoid *fludrocortisone* for postural hypotension (which may respond to elevation of the head of the bed). It can be combined with flurbiprofen and ephedrine hydrochloride (both unlicensed use)
- Anticholinergics, such as *propantheline*, for relief of gustatory sweating
- *Tetracycline* 250 mg (2 to 3 doses – unlicensed) for diarrhoea; otherwise, *codeine phosphate* is the best drug
- *Metoclopramide, domperidone* and *cisapride* for the treatment of gastroparesis
- The anti-muscarinic *ephedrine hydrochloride* (30 to 60 mg TDS, unlicensed) may offer effective relief for neuropathic oedema
- Several drugs for bladder and erectile dysfunction.

Although these treatments do not change the underlying disease process, they may improve quality of life.

Referral to secondary care

If the primary care team has no success, *referral* to either a diabetologist or a pain clinic is indicated. Some mononeuropathies caused by external compression (e.g. carpal tunnel) can be treated by *surgical decompression* with a good prognosis.

ERECTILE DYSFUNCTION

RATIONALE

There is a greater prevalence of erectile dysfunction in diabetics (AACE 2003), affecting up to 50% of those aged over 50 years, compared to 15–20% in those without diabetes (Marshall & Flyvbjerg 2006). In most cases of erectile dysfunction the causation is believed to be multifactorial. Age is the variable most strongly associated with erectile dysfunction (Feldman et al 1994).

AIM

The aim is to restore or compensate for sexual dysfunction in accordance with the patient's wishes.

EVALUATION

The causes of failure to achieve and maintain a satisfactory erection can include psychogenic or organic (i.e. vascular, neurogenic or endocrine) "abnormalities". Apart from diabetes, other potential causes need to be considered (Ralph et al 2000).

History

The history aims to define the dysfunction and to identify any possible contributory factors. If there is a partner, his or her presence is helpful. Relevant areas to question are:

Nature of the dysfunction

Is the problem a lack of tumescence or early collapse of erection or both? How long has it been going on, and did it start suddenly or gradually? Do spontaneous or early morning erections ever occur? Is libido normal and sexual stimulation present? Is there a problem with orgasm and ejaculation, and what is considered normal? Details of the current relationship, the partner's attitude and the couple's expectations. What remedies have been tried already?

Current medical history

It is useful to look for endocrine abnormalities (hair loss, gynaecomastia, weight gain and change in heat tolerance), vascular disease (exercise-related chest or leg pain) and neurological disorder (problems with sensation, co-ordination and motor function).

Past medical history

Enquire about pelvic surgery, radiotherapy or trauma, and psychiatric or psychological problems.

Medication

Many drugs can cause erectile dysfunction: thiazide diuretics, β-blockers, antidepressants, tranquillisers, anxiolytics and H2 antagonists.

Lifestyle

As well as smoking and alcohol, ask about recent major life changes and the use of recreational or bodybuilding drugs.

Information from the above should provide strong clues as to the origin of the dysfunction. Sudden onset, the presence of some erections, ejaculatory problems and major life events and/or psychological problems suggest a psychogenic cause, whereas gradual onset, no tumescence, the presence of risk factors, a past history of pelvic disease or treatment, certain medication or illicit drug use, smoking and heavy alcohol consumption suggest an organic cause.

Examination

Often examination can be limited to the genitalia, looking for anatomical abnormalities (e.g. retractability of the foreskin if present, hypospadias or fibrosis in the penile shaft), the presence of pubic hair, and any evidence of testicular atrophy. Either the history or this initial examination may indicate further examination, such as looking for the presence of secondary sexual characteristics (e.g. breasts, beard growth).

Investigations

Further investigations are indicated by the clinical findings. A free serum testosterone is the preferred screening investigation for suspected hypogonadism. Other investigations may be appropriate, such as thyroid function, prostate specific antigen and prolactin. Extensive endocrine investigations are usually unnecessary.

Interventions

Some patients may not be enthusiastic about medical intervention for erectile dysfunction. As a first step, optimising glycaemic control, encouraging smoking cessation and treating underlying causes (such as altering problem medication) may be helpful.

If the difficulty is thought to be psychogenic, then an exploration of the surrounding issues may identify the cause. Often performance anxiety and lack of self-confidence may be contributory. Sometimes offering an explanation, reassurance and clear unbiased information about treatment options, respecting patients' wishes, may be sufficient. However, referral for pyschosexual therapy may be indicated if simple measures do not work. If the waiting list is very long, other appropriate therapeutic interventions should be considered in the meantime.

Pharmacological options

Drug treatments for erectile dysfunction may be prescribed on the NHS only under certain circumstances. Diabetes mellitus is one of the allowable conditions, provided the prescription is endorsed "SLS". The maximum prescribable quantity on the NHS is one treatment per week, but there is no limit on private prescriptions as long as the medical indications, contraindications and cautions are respected. None of these should be prescribed where sexual activity is medically inadvisable.

The availability of phosphodiesterase type-5 inhibitors (PDE5) has revolutionised the treatment of erectile dysfunction. In the absence of contraindications, these agents are the current first-line pharmacological intervention.

Phosphodiesterase type-5 inhibitors

This class of drugs selectively inhibits phosphodiesterase 5, an enzyme that breaks down cyclic guanosine monophosphate (GMP), an intracellular second messenger that produces smooth muscle relaxation and maintains penile blood flow. These drugs have no effect on the libido and do not produce an erection in the absence of sexual stimulation. Although effective and well-tolerated in many, 30 to 35% of patients fail to respond (McMahon et al 2006).

There are currently three agents available: *sildenafil*, *tadalafil* and *vardenafil*. All are taken orally prior to sexual activity and can be quite effective. The maximum dose is one in 24 hours.

It is important to know their:

- *Contraindications*: severe hepatic impairment, hypotension (blood pressure <90/50 mmHg), recent stroke or myocardial infarction, unstable angina, hereditary degenerative retinal disorders and concurrent treatment with nitrates, nitric oxide donors and ritonavir [human immunodeficiency virus (HIV) protease inhibitor].
- *Cautions*: in anatomical penile deformity (e.g. angulation, cavernosal fibrosis, Peyronie's disease), conditions predisposing to priapism (e.g. sickle-cell disease, multiple myeloma or leukaemia) and concurrent treatment with cimetidine, erythromycin, ketoconazole, itraconazole and other HIV protease inhibitors.
- *Side effects*: headache, flushing, dyspepsia, vomiting, transient visual disturbances (which consist of a bluish tinge to white colours and last less than 20 minutes), raised intra-ocular pressure and nasal congestion.

Sildenafil was the first available oral drug for the treatment of erectile dysfunction. It should be taken 1 hour before sexual activity and has a duration of action of 4 hours. The usual starting dose is 50 mg, with a subsequent dose range of 25 to 100 mg (reduce dose in elderly, or hepatic or renal impairment). It should be used with caution in hepatic impairment (avoid if severe), renal impairment, bleeding disorders or active peptic ulcer. Serious cardiovascular events have been reported with sildenafil.

Tadalafil should be taken at least 30 minutes before sexual activity and has a duration of action of 24 hours. The usual starting dose is 10 mg, with a maximum dose of 20 mg. It should be used with caution in hepatic or renal impairment. In addition to the above, tadalafil is contraindicated in mild heart failure, uncontrolled arrhythmias and uncontrolled hypertension. Back pain and myalgia have been reported as side effects in addition to those listed above.

Vardenafil should be taken approximately 25 to 60 minutes before sexual activity, although the onset of effect may be delayed if taken with a fatty meal. Its cautions are similiar to sildenafil. It has a duration of action of 4 hours. Vardenafil's side effects also include, less commonly, drowsiness, hypertension, tachycardia, palpitation, back pain, myalgia and facial oedema.

When a PDE5 inhibitor fails, and before moving onto another treatment, the following should be considered:

- Incorrect use of drug or noncompliance. One study reported that 81% of men took sildenafil incorrectly and education solved the problem in 40% (Atiemo et al 2003). Other points are the need to allow sufficient time for the medication to work, and to avoid food and excessive alcohol that may delay or reduce drug absorption. Patients need to be warned that some may require up to six to eight doses before optimal response occurs (McCullough et al 2002).
- Dose optimisation. Doses do need to be titrated against response. Decreased responsiveness after repeated doses (tachyphylaxis) can occur.
- Switching agents. Although there are no comparative studies between the three agents, many patients will try another PDE5 inhibitor before moving onto other options.

Alprostadil
This agent is also known as prostaglandin E1. It is administered by intracavernosal injection (Caverject and Viridial) or intraurethral application (MUSE), both as a diagnostic test and as treatment for erectile dysfunction. The dose depends upon the preparation and response. The aim is to produce an erection lasting for 1 hour. Patients can self-administer after proper training (usually in an andrology clinic).

The contraindications are predisposition to prolonged erection, concurrent use of other agents for erectile dysfunction, and penile implants. The urethral application is contraindicated in urethral stricture, severe hypospadias, urethritis, balanitis and severe curvature. The side effects include penile pain, priapism (also a caution), local reactions at injection site, testicular pain and swelling.

Other treatments
Other currently licensed treatments should be considered if all of the above are contraindicated, unsuitable or ineffective. These include vacuum devices and penile prostheses. Referral to a suitable specialist clinic is usually advisable for these treatments.

Referral
Although most patients with erectile dysfunction can be managed safely and effectively in primary care, specialist referral should be considered to:

- A sex therapist
- A urologist if the patient has never had an erection and/or if there is a severe vascular problem and/or if the patient opts for an intervention beyond the practitioner's competence
- An endocrinologist if a hormone abnormality is found, although treatment may not restore potency.

INJECTION SITES

RATIONALE

Injecting insulin into abnormal subcutaneous tissue may affect the proportion that reaches the circulation and its timing, and, thus, affect glycaemic control. Also, the presence of infection at injection sites can affect health.

ASSESSMENT

The patient's insulin injection technique should be observed, and injection sites inspected for atrophy or infection.

INTERVENTIONS

Correct faults in the injection technique. Any infected sites should be treated with antibiotics or referred to the diabetic clinic. An earlier review may be necessary.

VASCULAR EMERGENCIES

MYOCARDIAL INFARCTION

Not only are type 2 diabetics at increased risk of suffering a CHD event, but, since the presentation may be atypical, there can be delays in their receiving appropriate medical care. It is not infrequent for an elderly diabetic to suffer no chest pain during a myocardial infarction. The only clues may be an ill patient, with some degree of cardiac dysfunction (abnormal pulse, hypotensive and/or signs of heart failure) and hyperglycaemia. Acute hospital admission may be needed to confirm diagnosis, or to deal with more complex management problems and social circumstances.

Following an acute myocardial infarction, patients with diabetes should be considered for intensive insulin treatment (currently under evaluation, but with promising results), as well as for the standard therapies of thrombolysis, beta blockers, antiplatelet therapy (aspirin, with the possible addition of clopidogrel) and ACE inhibitors (especially if there is any evidence of left ventricular dysfunction). Although all these therapies have their own side effects, the increased mortality of MI and the further risk of a second event justify a more aggressive approach in patients with diabetes.

LOWER-LIMB PROBLEMS

Evaluation and intervention are discussed in detail above. A loss of skin integrity that leads to an ulcer or gangrene is a potential emergency. To minimise the risk of permanent damage or limb loss, prevention or, if this fails, prompt appropriate management is essential.

VITREOUS HAEMORRHAGE

Vitreous haemorrhage arises usually from new retinal vessels. The patient often presents with acute visual loss. Immediate referral to an ophthalmologist is indicated.

CEREBROVAS\CULAR DISEASE

Cerebrovascular disease is the second most common cause of death in type 2 diabetics and can cause a range of devastating deficits:

- *Hemiplegia* is usually the result of atheromatous cerebrovascular disease, but it can be a rare transient manifestation of hypoglycaemia in patients on insulin
- Other *reversible focal neurological deficits* also usually result from atheromatous cerebrovascular disease, but can occur in the rare HONK
- *Convulsions* may result from structural cerebral damage caused by cerebrovascular disease, but can be triggered by hyperglycaemia if there is hyperosmolarity in susceptible patients
- *Cognitive impairment* may result from atherosclerotic dementia, but hyperglycaemia is also thought to produce psychological dysfunction. Better glycaemic control may improve cognition.

The primary care interventions for prevention of stroke include:

- Antiplatelet therapy, such as aspirin (if not contraindicated), although there is not yet any clear evidence that alternative antiplatelet regimens are more or less effective
- Blood pressure reduction (although no blood pressure reduction regimen has been shown to be superior to others)

and

- Cholesterol reduction (Lip et al 2003).

In addition to hypertension and increasing age, atrial fibrillation has been identified by the UKPDS as a major risk factor for stroke in type 2 diabetics (Davies et al 1999). As well as vigorous correction of other risk factors, control of rate (if cardioversion is not possible or successful) and anticoagulation should be considered, with aspirin as an alternative if anticoagulation is either contraindicated or unsuitable. Guidance on the optimal management of atrial fibrillation can be found in the latest edition of the British National Formulary, Section 2.3.1. Seeking a cardiology specialist opinion is often advisable.

► KEY POINTS

- The management of most diabetic complications includes both condition-specific interventions, and optimising glycaemic control and cardiovascular risk factors.

- Mydriatic retinal photography is the preferred screening method for diabetic retinopathy.

- The mainstays of treatment for diabetic retinopathy are the modification of cardiovascular risk and referral for laser photocoagulation and/or cataract removal.

- Screening for diabetic nephropathy should include estimating the urinary albumin (or protein)–creatinine ratio and glomerular filtration rate. The most important treatment is blood pressure lowering, usually by inhibition of the renin-angiotensin system.

- The diabetic foot is a group of syndromes in which neuropathy, ischaemia and infection lead to tissue breakdown, which results in morbidity. Up to 50% of ulcers and amputations can be prevented by prompt and effective interventions.

- High-risk feet or those with active disease require referral to a multidisciplinary foot care team.

- Diabetic neuropathy has diverse clinical manaifestations, but the most common are distal symmetric polyneuropathy and autonomic neuropathy.

- A variety of drugs, including tricyclic antidepressants and antiepilepsy, have a role to play in relieving neuropathic pain.

- The availability of phosphodiesterase type-5 inhibitors has revolutionised the treatment of erectile dysfunction, but up to one-third of men fail to respond to these drugs.

- Amongst the important diabetes complications, vascular events need to be included, such as myocardial infarction, lower limb gangrene, vitreous haemorrhage and cerebrovascular disease.

LIVING WITH DIABETES

OVERVIEW

MENTAL HEALTH

An individual with a chronic disease is more vulnerable to a range of psychological and psychiatric disorders. Depression and anxiety are commoner in diabetics than in the general population. The presence of complications further lowers the quality of life and increases the likelihood of depression. The interaction between mental health and diabetes can lead to a vicious cycle of worsening diabetic management and mental illness.

There are a number of studies showing that the prevalence of depression is greater in the diabetic population than in the nondiabetic population:

- One meta-analysis calculated the odds of depression in diabetics to be double that of nondiabetics. This did not differ by sex, type of diabetes, subject source, or assessment method. The prevalence of comorbid depression was significantly higher in diabetic women than in diabetic men. The paper also suggested that depression was clinically relevant in nearly one-third of patients with diabetes (Anderson et al 2001).
- In an Australian study, the prevalence of depression in the diabetic population was 24% compared to 17% in the nondiabetic population (Goldney et al 2004).
- In another meta-analysis, although the prevalence of comorbid depression was significantly higher in people with type 2 diabetes than those without (17.6% vs. 9.8%), diabetics (compared to non-diabetics) differed on variables known to be associated with an increased risk of depression and potential confounders were not always reported. More rigorous studies are required (Ali 2006).

This increased prevalence of depression among diabetics underpins the new QOF indicators added in 2006: all patients with diabetes and/or heart disease should be screened "on one occasion during the previous 15 months" for depression using the two standard screening questions:

- "During the last month, have you often been bothered by feeling down, depressed or hopeless?"
- "During the last month, have you often been bothered by having little interest or pleasure in doing things?"

A positive response to either question should be followed up by asking the patient if he wants help and a structured assessment of depression.

Interestingly, the evidence underpinning the new indicators has been challenged. A Cochrane review concluded "that routine feedback of the results of screening to clinicians results in a marginal increase in the rate of diagnosis of depression. However, patients' outcomes are not improved at 6–12 months as a consequence of screening". The review also concluded that the sceening test fails to meet the National Screening Committee's criteria for the test, the treatment and the screening programme (see Chapter 1) (Gilbody et al 2006).

From diagnosis, both health-care professionals and carers can play an important role in the mental health of diabetics:

- By providing adequate psychological support to enable patients to come to terms with their diabetes and to take increasing control of their disease, one of the aims of care. Diabetes can cause psychological distress, separate from mental illness.
- By early recognition and appropriate management of mental illness, which can affect diabetes care adversely. Involvement of the local mental-health team or liaison psychiatrist may be necessary. Depression with biological features usually requires pharmacological therapy, preferably with a selective serotonin reuptake inhibitor (SSRI), which may improve glycaemic control (Lustman et al 2000).
- By recognising the full range of nonmedical (e.g. social, financial) factors that can affect patients, and by accepting that in the patients' minds these may have precedence over diabetes and other medical problems – solving other problems may be the most effective way to improve both diabetes-related and mental health.

Cognitive behaviour therapy is also useful in treating depression, but is less effective in diabetics with complications (Lustman et al 1988).

DRIVING

LEGAL PROVISIONS

The current guidelines are regularly updated and found on the Driver and Vehicle Licensing Agency's (DVLA) website: *http://www.dvla.gov.uk/at_a_glance/ch3_diabetes.htm*). This also provides contact details for the DVLA.

The Road Traffic Acts require that diabetics (irrespective of treatment) who are either applicants or driving licence holders must notify the DVLA of their condition and of any problems or diabetes complications that develop that may affect the safety of driving. Failure to inform the DVLA is now a criminal offence. For medico-legal reasons, health-care professionals should document in the medical records that they have advised the patient to notify the DVLA. GPs may be contacted by a medical officer from the DVLA with a request for further information (usually a DIAB3 form), such as details about glycaemic control (particularly the risk of hypoglycaemia), visual problems and any limb problems.

The medical standards for licence entitlement (more stringent for Group 1 than Group 2 licences) include:

1. *Adequate visual acuity* with or without correction, equivalent of Snellen chart 6/12
2. *Minimum visual field* of at least 120° on the horizontal, with no significant defect in the binocular field
3. *Adequate awareness of hypoglycaemia.* In addition, if frequent episodes impair driving, then driving "must cease" until adequate control is regained
4. If *limb disability* is present, driving is possible in both static and progressive or relapsing disorders, but vehicle modification may be needed and the DVLA notified
5. *Absence of significant symptoms*, e.g. sudden disabling attacks of giddiness or fainting or impaired psychomotor or cognitive function.

Group 1 (ordinary) licence holders and applicants on insulin are granted a licence up to 3 years. On renewal they are required to make a self-declaration that may lead to medical enquiries. Those treated with diet and tablets or diet alone are permitted to hold a licence valid to 70 years of age, subject to the conditions and the need to report any change to insulin treatment. For Group 1 (ordinary) licence holders and applicants, a questionnaire (Diabetic 1) needs to be completed (downloadable: *http://www.dvla. gov.uk/drivers/dmed1_ files/pdf/diab1.pdf*).

Since 1991, diabetics on insulin have been banned from applying for and renewing thereafter a *Group 2* (bus, coach and large goods vehicle driver) licence. Diabetics on diet alone or diet and tablet treatment are permitted to hold a Group 2 licence, subject to the absence of any relevant disability and to not being on insulin. Also, drivers with insulin-treated diabetes should not drive emergency vehicles, due to "… the difficulties for an individual, regardless of whether they may appear to have exemplary glycaemic control, in adhering to the monitoring processes required when responding to an emergency situation" (DVLA 2006).

Insulin is a drug within the meaning of the Road Traffic Act 1988, and a driver "in control of a motor vehicle" with symptoms of hypoglycaemia runs the risk of being charged with driving under the influence of drugs. To avoid this and to correctly manage a hypoglycaemic episode:

- The vehicle must be stopped (with ignition switched off) and in a safe place
- The driver not seated behind the steering wheel
- The low blood glucose level should be corrected (with either a suitable source of sugar or glucagon)

  and

- The journey should not be resumed until recovery is complete. This may take 15 or more minutes and the blood glucose level should be checked first.

INSURANCE

If an insurance company asks about diabetes, then the applicant must inform the company if he is diabetic. Failure to do so and also to notify the DVLA can invalidate cover in the event of a claim.

Since the Disability Discrimination Act (1995) came into effect at the end of 1996, insurers can refuse or charge more for cover *only* with evidence of an increased risk of making a claim. However, because most evidence available about diabetic drivers indicates that they pose no higher risk than nondiabetic drivers, many insurance companies no longer ask about diabetes when cover is applied for.

Some companies, who base their risk assessment on their experience of drivers with diabetes, may still refuse cover or impose special terms or charge an increased premium if their statistics "show" a higher risk. When this happens, it is worth challenging the insurer, especially if the applicant's diabetes is stable and well controlled. It is always worth shopping around for quotes from a number of insurers, as premiums can vary considerably.

MEDICAL PROBLEMS THAT MAY AFFECT DRIVING

Patients and professionals need to be aware of the following that can affect driving:

- *Visual problems* arise usually from either retinopathy or cataract. Incorrectable deterioration of visual acuity, loss of peripheral visual field through widespread ablative retinal photocoagulation, may also result in loss of fitness to drive.
- *Hypoglycaemia* (discussed above).
- Neurological and/or vascular deficit may result in severe *damage to the feet* (leading to ulcers, or even amputation), and so also results in loss of fitness to drive.
- *Arterial disease* may result in cardiovascular and/or cerebrovascular disability, which affects fitness to drive.
- *Alcohol* lowers blood glucose levels, increasing the risk of hypoglycaemia in those on insulin or certain oral medication. A hypo may look like drunkenness; if the breath smells of alcohol this could heighten suspicion. Hyperglycaemia, even in the presence of ketones, will not affect a breathalyser machine.

IMMUNISATIONS

QOF ◄
DM18

Influenza and pneumonia are common, preventable infectious diseases associated with high mortality and morbidity in people with chronic diseases, such as diabetes. There are limited data on the morbidity and mortality of influenza and pneumococcal pneumonia specifically in diabetics. Safe and effective vaccines are available that can greatly reduce the risk of serious complications from these diseases. Unless contraindicated, the DoH recommends immunisation against influenza and pneumococcal pneumonia in all individuals with diabetes.

EMPLOYMENT

Diabetes UK has produced a useful booklet, *Employment and diabetes*.

FINDING A JOB

Diabetics on insulin are still not allowed to be in the following occupations:

- Driving either a heavy goods or public service or emergency vehicle
- Certain jobs in the Armed Forces, such as front-line troops and pilots
- Working offshore, such as on an oil rig or cruise ship
- Working at heights
- Being a jockey.

Since October 2004, blanket bans have been lifted for diabetics joining the police, fire and ambulance services, but applicants need to demonstrate that their diabetes is well controlled (with hypo-awareness), regularly monitored, and free of complications. The minimum levels of physical and mental fitness are still necessary for all applicants.

Any diabetic is entitled to be considered for any employment for which he is otherwise qualified. UK (via the Disability Discrimination Act) and European legislation offer protection against discrimination in employment against individuals with a medical condition such as diabetes. Due to a lack of up-to-date knowledge about diabetes, employers may fear that a diabetic poses a potential safety risk to the employer and/or the public. Most diabetics can manage their condition so that there is minimal risk of incapacitation from problems such as hypoglycaemia (ADA 2007). Employers need to consider whether the individual's qualifications and medical circumstances (the condition, its treatment and any specific risks or problems) can be matched to the job specification. The Disability Rights Commission provides useful information for both employers and workers with long-term conditions such as diabetes.

Changing working hours

Working shifts can increase the risk of developing either metabolic syndrome or type 2 diabetes (Knutsson 2003). Altering working hours, such as changing shifts or working overtime, can disrupt eating and sleeping patterns in people with pre-existing diabetes, and may lead to a worsening of glycaemic control, particularly if the rotation pattern is rapid. Increased physical activity can affect blood glucose levels, and may require adjustments in calorific intake and treatment to maintain reasonable glycaemic control. Physically demanding work at unexpected times increases the risk of hypoglycaemia.

The following advice may be useful to diabetics working odd hours:

- Make sure meals or snacks are available
- Try to arrange meal breaks to be at set times
- Have a fast-acting carbohydrate snack readily available at all times in case of hypoglycaemia
- Monitor blood glucose levels more frequently
- Ensure that work colleagues are aware of diagnosis of diabetes, especially if working alone.

If on insulin, then it is sensible to use a newer prolonged-acting insulin (insulins glargine or detemir) as the basal insulin. These have the advantages of only being administered once daily and at the same time of day irrespective of the work pattern. Rapid-acting analogues (insulins lispro, aspart or glulisine) can then be administered to cover unpredictable and variable mealtimes. Where possible, patients should aim to time meals at 4 to 5 hour intervals, with snacks if required, and to keep to consistent quantities and types of food.

Adjustments to dosages, type and/or timing of insulin are usually necessary when working shifts, although administering insulin can usually be delayed 1 to 2 hours without significantly affecting diabetic control. This may be sufficient to cover an afternoon shift. If extra food is consumed later in the day, an appropriate increase in the later insulin dose may be needed. Major changes, such as moving to and from night shifts, require careful planning of food intake (more during the shift) and insulin administration, and patients may seek professional advice.

INTERCURRENT ILLNESS

The stress of illness can produce transient insulin resistance and worsen glycaemic control; even if there is little or no calorific intake. Patients treated with diet only or on oral medication may temporarily require insulin.

The following advice should be given to diabetics who become unwell:

- Keeping testing blood (or urinary) glucose regularly throughout the day
- Do **not** stop basal insulin, although the dose may need adjusting
- Try to drink plenty of fluids (water, sugary fluids or milk) and, if possible, eat soups, snacks or biscuits to maintain a calorific intake
- If unable to keep anything down or if urine test for ketones becomes positive or if having trouble controlling blood glucose, seek medical help. Hospital admission may be necessary more often in diabetics to treat infection and/or correct dehydration.

TRAVEL

Diabetics do and should be able to travel. They need to observe the same precautions as the rest of the population, but also to make their own arrangements to reduce the risk of diabetes complications and emergencies. Constant perfect glycaemic control is not an absolute necessity, but the extremes of hypoglycaemia and hyperglycaemia should be avoided.

Pre-travel planning is essential and involves obtaining essential information, ensuring current optimal diabetic management and having in place all the necessary arrangements. Health-care professionals and organisations, such as Diabetes UK and the NHS Scotland (on its website, *www.fitfortravel.scot.nhs.uk*), can provide useful information.

DOCUMENTATION

Patients should wear or carry some form of medical identification, such as a bracelet or necklace. In this period of heightened concerns about travel security, diabetic travellers should carry a practice- or hospital-headed letter from their practice that lists their medical problems, repeat medication and supplies, and confirms that their medication and devices (including needles and syringes) are required and appropriate for their personal therapeutic needs, and needs to be carried on the plane. This letter should be shown at check-in and at Customs. It may also be useful if seeking medical attention abroad.

INSURANCE

It is prudent to obtain adequate travel insurance and to carry the necessary sickness insurance forms in case of illness abroad. It is important to check that "pre-existing conditions" are not excluded.

Holders of the European Health Insurance Card (EHIC), which has replaced the old form E111, are entitled to reduced-cost or sometimes free essential medical treatment in all countries in the European Economic Area and Switzerland. Travellers with chronic conditions, including diabetes, may also be covered for treatment. This card should be obtained prior to departure, either online, via: *http://www.dh.gov.uk/PolicyAndGuidance/HealthAdviceForTravellers/GettingTreatmentAroundTheWorld/fs/*, or by telephoning 0845 606 2030, or from a Post Office.

It is advisable to also obtain travel insurance. Among the options available, Diabetes UK Insurance Services offers its own products, available online from May 2006 (see Diabetes UK website and follow links).

VACCINATIONS

Diabetics are advised to have the necessary vaccinations well in advance of departure, as these may cause a transient disturbance of glycaemic control.

PACKING

Diabetics should carry sufficient and suitably packed supplies of their medication (including either glucagon or glucose tablets to treat hypoglycaemia), supplies, testing equipment, and documentation for their trip. If possible, prescription medications should be kept in their original containers, and other items (such as syringes, alcohol swabs and test strips) should be packed in plastic bags with zipper-type seals. Any glass items should be wrapped carefully in socks or placed between soft clothing during transport.

If flying, then medication, supplies, fast- and slow-acting carbohydrates, and documentation should be packed in carry-on luggage, rather than stowed. Extra quantities should be taken in case of delays, mishaps or if further supplies are unlikely to be available at the destination.

Insulin must be kept out of direct sunlight and should always be kept cool, either in a cool bag or some form of cool storage, although open insulin vials retain their potency at temperate room temperatures for up to 1 month. Insulin should *not* be kept in car glove compartments (too hot) or in checked luggage (it will end up in the plane's hold where it might freeze. After defrosting, it is likely to be less active).

MEDICATION

In a few countries insulin is not available in U100 strength, but in U40. If patients switch to U40 insulin abroad, to ensure the correct dose they should also use U40 syringes and so avoid any mixture with U100.

MODIFYING TREATMENT REGIMENS

In aiming to avoid hypoglycaemia or marked hyperglycaemia, diabetics are advised to run their blood sugars slightly higher than normal, particularly during long journeys.

Travelling by plane

If the journey is by plane, diabetic control can be adversely affected. Most short flights should not cause much difficulty. However, on long flights, delays and uncertain meal times can pose problems.

When booking the flight ticket, the airline may be able to provide information about meal times. If possible, diabetics should choose an in-flight meal that contains complex carbohydrates, such as pasta or rice. The vegetarian option may be a more likely source of this type of carbohydrate than the "diabetic" meal, which may contain little or no carbohydrate.

If on oral medication, diabetics may wish to transfer to a shorter-acting sulphonylurea during the journey.

Changing time zones

Travelling across time zones and eating different foods at unpredictable times both require adjustment of treatment regimes, particularly if on insulin. Some of the principles used for diabetics who observe fasting during Ramadan may apply. It may be necessary to reduce the dose of basal insulin to keep blood sugars "ticking over" and to administer rapid-acting insulin with meals.

- When travelling west, the day of travel becomes longer. If the time difference is five or more hours, then an extra meal may be needed, covered either by rapid- or short-acting insulin or by a higher or extra dose of oral medication.
- When travelling east, the day of travel becomes shorter. If the time difference is five or more hours, the day may be too short to fit in all the usual meals. If a meal is omitted, then it may not be necessary to administer the short- or rapid-acting insulin or to take the oral medication that normally covers it.

When away from home

High temperatures can increase insulin absorption. To avoid hypoglycaemia, when travelling or exercising in hot climates, a reduction in the insulin dose may be necessary. In hot climates, insulin needs to be stored either in a refrigerator (avoiding freezing) or an air-conditioned room. When out and about, insulin should be carried in a cool bag.

If ill, insulin and/or oral hypoglycaemic medication should never be stopped, even if the patient is unable to take solid foods. Diabetics should be prepared to manage vomiting and diarrhoea when abroad, but should seek local medical help if symptoms persist or if they become ill.

OTHER PRECAUTIONS

Drinking only bottled water, avoiding salads and being careful about hygiene levels in restaurants are sensible precautions. Diabetics need to take on holiday comfortable, well-fitting shoes in case their feet swell in hot weather. They should avoid going barefoot, particularly on hot sand. As with nondiabetic travellers, appropriate emergency medication should be carried.

PREGNANCY AND GESTATIONAL DIABETES

Pregnancy in women with previously diagnosed type 2 diabetes is a different condition from gestational diabetes mellitus. However, many components of management are the same for both conditions.

PREGNANCY IN WOMEN WITH PREVIOUSLY DIAGNOSED TYPE 2 DIABETES

Pregnancy is associated with increased risks in both type 1 and type 2 diabetes. Major congenital malformations remain the leading cause of mortality and serious morbidity in infants of mothers with type 2 diabetes (ADA 2007). The development of congenital malformations of major organs correlates with elevated HbA1c levels, both at conception and during the first 8 weeks of pregnancy.

With the increasing prevalence and earlier onset of type 2 diabetes, it is possible that primary care will encounter type 2 diabetics who conceive and become pregnant. However, the lead in the management of these women should be a specialist obstetric-endocrine clinic to achieve best outcomes.

MANAGEMENT

Monitoring should be undertaken for other known risks, and managed according to best practice.

Pre-conception

It is at this time that primary care can play a valuable role. There is evidence that foetal malformations can be reduced or prevented by careful management of diabetes before conception. However, many women with diabetes who conceive, have unplanned pregnancies, making it difficult to provide pre-conception care.

Type 2 diabetics are less likely to receive pre-conception counselling than those with type 1 diabetes. Care should aim to address the following areas:

- Weight management. Prior to conception, the woman should aim to achieve a BMI of less than $27 \, \text{kg/m}^2$ weight loss may be indicated.

- Glycaemic control should be optimal at conception, aiming for a "reasonable" HbA1c (trying to avoid sustained hyperglycaemia). If on oral hypoglycaemic medication or if HbA1c is raised, then the patient should be started on insulin prior to conception.
- Diet should be low in fat, high in complex carbohydrates and high in dietary fibre.
- Increased physical activity can be encouraged.
- Certain drugs commonly prescribed to women with diabetes should be stopped prior to conception: statins, ACE or ARB, metformin (but see below) and acarbose.

Ante-natal care

Maintaining optimal glycaemic control is the key to achieving the best maternal and neonatal outcomes. The specialist obstetric-endocrine clinic team may include not just an obstetrician and diabetologist, but also a dietician and a diabetes specialist nurse. However, primary health-care professionals often play a supporting role.

For optimal glycaemic control during pregnancy, the suggested target capillary plasma glucose levels are:

- Before meals: 4.4–6.1 mmol/l
- 2 hours after meals: less than 8.6 mmol/l (DoH/Diabetes UK 2005).

Folic acid

As in GDM, pregnant diabetics are at increased risk of having babies with neural tube defects (NTDs). They should be prescribed (as this dose is prescription-only medicine) a daily supplement of 5 mg of folic acid before conceiving and during the first 12 weeks of pregnancy.

Diet

The timing of meals should be to ensure a regular and adequate caloric intake throughout the day; however, calorific intake needs to be monitored to prevent excessive weight gain (greater than 9 kg). Women are advised to avoid concentrated sweets. The diet should also contain adequate nutrients to meet the needs of pregnancy. Obese women should avoid daytime snacks and restrict their calorific intake.

Glycaemic medication

To achieve good glycaemic control and current practice is that insulin should replace oral medication, although no insulin is actually licensed for use during pregnancy (DoH/Diabetes UK 2005). The dosage, type and regimen should be tailored to the needs of the individual. If on an established insulin regimen, including analogue insulin, then change is not always necessary; however, there is no evidence for the safety of insulin glargine in pregnancy. It is likely that basal (intermediate- or prolonged-acting) insulin will be needed, in addition to prandial (rapid- or short-acting) insulin before meals.

However, it may be possible to use certain oral hypoglycaemic agents in pregnancy without increasing the risk of congenital malformations occurring. In a recent review, there was no difference found in outcomes between pregnant women treated with metformin and "controls" (Hughes & Rowan 2006). There is also evidence to suggest that the level of glycaemia at conception and subsequently correlates with the development of anomalies, and not the use of certain oral agents.

Hypoglycaemia

The risk of hypoglycaemia is greater in early pregnancy. Those close to the woman should be instructed in the recognition, management and treatment of hypoglycaemia. If a woman loses her hypoglycaemia awareness during pregnancy, she should be advised not to drive.

Physical activity

Although there is insufficient evidence to recommend, or advise against, diabetic pregnant women enrolling in exercise programmes (Ceysens et al 2006), moderate exercise after meals should be encouraged, but women need to be cautioned about hypoglycaemia.

Blood pressure

Women with type 2 diabetes are more at risk of developing hypertension during pregnancy.

Fundoscopy

Women with existing diabetic retinopathy are at increased risk of the retinopathy progressing during their pregnancy. Thus, more frequent eye screening may be necessary. Detailed retinal screening is advised in both the first and third trimesters (DoH/Diabetes UK 2005). If new vessel formation (and, occasionally, macular oedema) is found, then treatment must be started promptly.

Labour and delivery

If delivery occurs before 36 weeks' gestation, then corticosteroids (betamethasone) should be administered to prevent neonatal respiratory distress syndrome. Additional insulin usually needs to be given to prevent severe maternal hyperglycaemia.

With good glycaemic control, and in the absence of significant diabetic or other complications, it may be possible to prolong pregnancy to 39 weeks to achieve a vaginal delivery, although this may vary according to local policy. The rate of delivery by caesarean section is higher than in women without diabetes. Women need to be assessed at 38 weeks' gestation to plan for the delivery. Delivery takes place in a consultant-led unit, with neonatal intensive care available.

Postpartum

Immediately after delivery of the placenta, maternal insulin sensitivity improves. If on insulin prior to pregnancy, then the dose usually returns to that at pre-conception.

Breast feeding

Breast milk contains lactose: every time a woman feeds her baby, her blood glucose level will fall. To help prevent hypoglycaemic episodes, women who are breast feeding may need to reduce their insulin dose (by up to 30%) and/or increase their intake of starchy foods. This will vary between women.

GESTATIONAL DIABETES MELLITUS (GDM)

This is defined as diabetes mellitus with onset or first recognition during pregnancy. Pregnancy can act as a metabolic stress test for diabetes, resulting in gestational diabetes developing in those who "fail". The condition should be regarded as heterogeneous, as women who develop it may be either obese, hyperinsulinaemic and insulin-resistant or thin and relatively insulin-deficient.

Much of the management of women with GDM should be the same as for pregnant women with diabetes previously diagnosed.

Epidemiology

Incidence
GDM is thought to occur in 1–3% of pregnancies, but this incidence may be higher in certain populations such as Indo-Asians, Pacific Islanders and Native Americans.

Risk factors
The characteristics of women with an increased or high risk of developing GDM include:

- Previous history of GDM
- Marked obesity
- Strong family history of diabetes mellitus
- Glycosuria present.

Once pregnancy is confirmed, these women should be screened as soon as possible.

Diagnosis

Criteria
The diagnostic criteria for GDM are the same as for other diabetes. However, the ADA's clinical practice recommendations do appear to have lower blood glucose thresholds for the diagnosis, following a 100 g (not 75 g) glucose load modified OGTT.

Screening
Pregnant women should be screened for diabetes. Diabetes UK recommends performing an OGTT, using a 75 g glucose load for the challenge, in women with "random" plasma glucose levels greater than 6.1 mmol/l fasting or 7.0 mmol/l within 2 hours of food. The diagnostic criteria for GDM, as defined by the World Health Organization (WHO), are levels of venous plasma glucose greater than 7.0 mmol/l fasting (same as normal diabetic criterion) **or** 7.8 mmol/l 2 hours post challenge (in the impaired glucose tolerance range of "standard" diabetes).

The ADA recommends performing an OGTT using a 100 g glucose load for the challenge, since using a 75 g load has not been "as well validated for detection of at-risk infants or mothers" (ADA 2007). The ADA diagnostic criteria for the 100 g glucose load OGTT are **two** or more plasma glucose values at or above:

- 5.3 mmol/l (fasting – 8–14 hours without calorific intake)
- 10 mmol/l (at 1 hour)
- 8.6 mmol/l (at 2 hours)
- 7.8 mmol/l (at 3 hours).

Management

Ante-natal

This is similar to management of pregnancy in women with pre-existing diabetes. Specific points to make about GDM include:

- Glycaemic control – basal insulin may not be required. However, small doses of short- or rapid-acting insulin need to be administered if the 2 hour post-prandial blood glucose level rises above 6.6 mmol/l. This level should be checked regularly, either by the patient or in clinic.
- Proteinuria and blood pressure – since women with GDM are at greater risk of developing hypertension, they should have urinalysis performed (checking for protein) and blood pressure recorded in clinic.

Labour and delivery

Delivery by term is recommended. Gestation more than 42 weeks should be avoided. The management of labour and delivery is the same as for women who were diabetic prior to conception.

Post-partum

Insulin can usually be stopped. Women should have a fasting blood glucose checked post-partum. If it is greater than 6.0 mmol/l, then a 75 g OGTT should be done at 6 weeks.

Rate of progression to type 2 diabetes mellitus

Women who have had GDM, but then return to normal glucose homeostasis, need to be advised of the increased risk of developing GDM in subsequent pregnancies and of type 1 or 2 diabetes in later life. However, this risk can be reduced by improving lifestyle: better diet, increased physical activity and optimising weight management.

CULTURAL ASPECTS OF DIABETES CARE

GENERAL POINTS

Many practices in the UK, particularly those in urban areas, look after ethnically, spiritually and culturally diverse populations. These factors can affect both the diagnosis (especially if using a bio-social model) and how health care is delivered.

Irrespective of culture, clear effective communication remains an essential part of the interaction between professional and patient. If English is not the patient's first language, it must not be assumed that the patient has English proficiency. The professional should be prepared to invest extra time and care in eliciting the necessary information and in ensuring that any messages given are understood (avoid jargon, do not sound condescending and ask the patient to relate what has just been said).

In Afro-Asian culture, a greater emphasis is placed on physical symptoms than on psychological ones, and there may be a greater expectation upon the doctor to make a diagnosis without a full assessment, and to provide a prescription rather than advice. Many Asians may feel that the diagnosis of diabetes is a stigma and consider the disease to be contagious. Many Afro-Asian patients may be reluctant to answer questions about their life and family histories. Eye contact may be poor. If a family attends, the husband or senior male figure often speaks on the patient's behalf. In contrast to the English sequence of "vision, hearing and touch", other cultures may prefer the sequence of "touch, hearing and vision". Afro-Asian patients may prefer to be examined by a professional of the same gender.

Many Afro-Asian diabetics use various types of traditional and/or herbal medicines regularly, even if they are taking conventional therapeutic medicines. Karela or guard is a recognised insulin-like substance.

DELIVERY OF DIABETES CARE TO ETHNIC MINORITIES

QOF◄
Record 21

A collective term used for this group of individuals is black and minority ethnic (BME), although it is important to remember that this is not a homogeneous population. In the GMS contract, practices are now expected to record the ethnic origin of all newly registered patients.

Costs
The UK Asian Diabetes Study (UKADS) estimated the annual costs for South Asian patients to be £365 per patient in 2004 (O'Hare et al 2004), higher than the UKPDS estimate of £264 in 1998. This higher cost includes the extra input of additional diabetes specialist nurses for this population. Further research is needed to determine the cost-effectiveness of "culturally sensitive" initiatives.

Lifestyle
Adopting a healthy lifestyle is important in diabetes management, irrespective of culture or ethnicity. The delivery of health education needs to be tailored to the social and cultural context.

Traditional South Asian cuisine often has a higher fat and sugar content. The use of ghee (clarified butter) is more "atherogenic" than standard butter. Traditional Indian sweets and popular snacks have both high fat and sugar content. Change may be difficult, since food is an important part of social life for many South Asian people; avoiding traditional foods may lead to "isolation". South Asians living in the UK tend to eat less fruit and vegetables than other groups (British Heart Foundation 2001).

Other aspects of lifestyle relevant to cardiovascular risk include:

- *Smoking*. South Asian men, particularly Bangladeshis, are more likely to smoke than white men, but smoking rates in South Asian women are lower than in their white counterparts (British Heart Foundation 2001).
- *Physical activity*. South Asian women may be reluctant to attend exercise classes unless single-sex facilities are available.
- *Alcohol*. Intake is often lower in South Asians, except in some Sikhs who may be heavy drinkers of spirits. Even though alcohol is prohibited by some religions, its consumption, and even abuse, may still occur.

Other customs that may be relevant to diabetes include:

- *Betel chewing* is common, particularly among adult Asians. Betel contains several active substances, and is a source of vitamin C, calcium and iron. Excessive use can lead to the development of stone in bladder, kidney or gall bladder. The tobacco chewed in betel is carcinogenic.
- *Hookla smoking* of tobacco leaves or paste is a common practice among Asian adults, particularly Bangladeshis.
- *Bathing* – some Asian patients take showers instead of baths, since it is unacceptable to sit in bathwater.

Alternative medications

In South Asian communities, herbs and herbal medicines are used frequently. The herb *karela* is used for its blood-glucose-lowering properties. Herbal preparations, particularly those bought in India and Pakistan, may have active ingredients that include sulphonylureas.

Language

Many members of the BME community living in the UK, especially of the older generation who were born abroad, speak little or no English. Some of these individuals have limited literacy in their own language. Both can affect communication. Individuals belonging to ethnic minorities are more likely to report gaps in their knowledge of diabetes (Audit Commission 2000). Written material in the appropriate language may be of less valuable than audio-visual material or the use of group work with a leader fluent in the language and aware of relevant culture and health beliefs. Locally organized events and days may also reach and help more isolated members of the South Asian community. Diabetes UK provides a range of well-presented materials (including leaflets and videos) in foreign languages and is involved in a variety of initiatives to support both patients and health professionals. Further details are available on its website: *www.diabetes.org.uk*.

Access to medical care

An important issue for BME individuals, and not just those with diabetes, is gaining access to appropriate medical care. In addition to language, different health beliefs and lifestyle (listed above), other factors that may have an adverse effect on this group obtaining care include poor knowledge of available services, social deprivation, lack of education, unemployment, lack of access to transport and differences in willingness to seek professional help.

Other support
The National Diabetes Support Team has set up an internet forum aimed at providing professionals with a place to ask for and exchange information to meet the health-care needs of BME individuals (online access: *http://www.diabetes.nhs.uk/forum/forum.asp?ForumID=5*).

___

ISLAM

Islam is a religion with a fundamental creed whose adherents (Muslims) come from various ethnic groups. Muslims are forbidden strictly to drink alcohol and to eat pork. Alternatives to porcine insulin and to tablets or capsules that contain gelatine must be provided.

Ramadan
Maintaining glycaemic control during Ramadan may be challenging.

Description
Ramadan is the ninth lunar month in the Islamic calendar year (starts 10 days earlier each year), during which no food or drink should be consumed between dawn and sunset. Fasting is obligatory for all healthy Muslim adults. Although certain groups, including ill people, are exempt from fasting, many diabetics may choose to fast. Diabetics controlled on diet alone should be able to fast with few problems.

Longer gaps between meals and greater amounts of food consumed during these meals may produce large fluctuations in blood glucose levels in diabetics who fast. It is worth knowing if patients have had previous experience of fasting and whether they are prepared to break the fast if hypoglycaemia occurs.

Diet
There are usually two meals, *Iftar* when the day's fast has finished, and *Sehri* before the next fast begins (this may be at a very early hour). Patients may consume large quantities of sugary fluids, carbohydrate-rich meals and fried food during these meals.

The following may help to optimise glycaemia:

- Limit the quantity of sweet foods at Iftar.
- Fill up on starchy foods, such as basmati rice, chapati or naan.
- Include fruit, vegetables, lentil and yoghurt in both meals.
- Delay Sehri to its proper time just before sunrise, rather than earlier near midnight, in order to spread out energy intake more evenly.
- Choose sugar-free drinks to quench thirst. Avoid adding sugar to drinks.
- Limit the quantity of fried foods.

Consuming the traditional rich foods associated with Ramadan and the religious festival *Eid-u-fir* risks weight gain. Advising total avoidance of these foods is counterproductive. Success is more likely if patients are helped to make healthy eating choices, limiting the quantities consumed of these rich foods, not just at Ramadan, but throughout the year.

Oral medication

Metformin
The risk of hypoglycaemia is low if on metformin monotherapy. Metformin should be taken at the end of fast to cover the period of eating, but consider reducing the dose or stopping if the patient feels unwell.

Sulphonylurea
If on glibenclamide, change to a quicker-acting sulphonylurea, e.g. tolbutamide or glipizide, to be taken once daily before Iftar. Glimepride is usually safe at a reduced dose to allow for its longer duration of action.

Post-prandial glucose regulators
Repaglinide is a useful alternative to a sulphonylurea when fasting because of its short duration of action.

Glitazones
The risk of hypoglycaemia is low with these agents. Although the timing does not need to be changed during Ramadan, the dosage may need to be reduced if the calorific and fat intake is lower.

Insulin

It may be inadvisable for some patients on insulin to fast, particularly if control is poor. If fasting, then insulin should usually not be stopped. Support and guidance is often needed to help people to adjust their insulin doses safely.

The following guidance may be useful:

- Avoid pre-mixed insulins during fasting. However, if the patient insists, then reduce the dose given at Sehri.
- Consider using lower-dose glargine or detemir as the basal insulin to reduce risk of hypoglycaemia during fast.
- Rapid-acting insulins are useful, as their short duration of action covers mealtimes with lower risk of hypoglycaemia during the fast or at night.
- Resting during the fasting period may help to avoid low blood glucose levels.

Hajj

Adult Muslims are obliged to make a pilgrimage to sacred areas in and around Mecca at least once in their lifetime, known as Hajj. Hajj can be physically gruelling, as it requires the pilgrim to walk for distances in heat under a strong sun.

Diabetics need to prepare carefully and take extra precautions. Among the points to consider are good-quality footwear, adequate hydration, insulin storage, correct immunisations (meningitis vaccination is now required following an outbreak, and hepatitis B is a potential risk if the pilgrim intends to have his head shaved by a barber using a communal razor) and adequate health insurance.

HINDUISM

Although Hinduism is a religion, it has many strands whose beliefs and customs are rather more diverse than in religions such as Islam. The vast majority of Hindus are of South Asian ethnicity.

Food

Food plays an important part in many Hindu's lives. Many Hindus are vegetarian, but even if meat is eaten, beef is not as cows are sacred. Foods with a high fat content are often consumed: sweets are frequently eaten and full cream milk is commonly used to make puddings. Sweets and rich fried food are often shared or exchanged.

Festivals

Most are characterised by many festivals that may involve fasting and feasting, and can last from 1–9 days. Erratic eating patterns can play havoc with glycaemic control. The three important Hindu festivals that may involve a change in eating patterns are:

- *Diwali* (festival of lights), which is celebrated by feasting.
- *Navrati* (celebrates death of demon Ravana by Rama), marked by fasting and dancing that may increase the risk of hypoglycaemia.
- *Holi* (festival of colours), marked by a single day of fasting.

Often these festivals can lead to overindulgence in foods with high carbohydrate and/or high saturated fat content.

SIKHISM

Sikhism originated from Hinduism, but has its own identity as a religion. Like Hindus, Sikhs do not eat beef. Many are vegetarians. Although alcohol is forbidden, high consumption and abuse does occur.

A Sikh temple (known as *Gurudhwara*) will serve free vegetarian meals with chipattis (with a high starch and fibre content) daily. Desserts are made with full cream milk, dry nuts and sugar. *Karah* is made with ghee (melted butter), dry nuts and full cream milk, and is served to visitors to a Sikh temple.

The Sikh festival *Diwali* includes distribution of sweets in its celebrations.

When undertaking a dietary assessment of a Sikh patient with diabetes, it is useful to enquire how much of the above food items are consumed.

JUDAISM

Although Judaism has a fundamental creed, Jews will vary in their level of adherence and may belong to different sects.

Kosher meat is like halal meat for Muslims. The killing of the animal must be performed so that the rabbi present at the time can give the seal of approval (known as *kashrut*). Orthodox Jews do not eat meat from pigs or animals with cloven hooves, nor shellfish. They are forbidden to eat meat and dairy products together or to use the same cutlery and crockery for these two groups of food.

Animal insulin could be prohibited under these rules, but Judaism does allow exemptions if adherence could be life threatening.

Jewish holy days or festivals include:

- *Yom Kippur,* the Day of Atonement, which involves fasting from sunset until an hour after sunset the following day. Children under 13, pregnant women and those with health problems are exempt from fasting.
- *Rosh Hashannah,* the Jewish New Year, is often celebrated with delicacies including honey cake.
- *Passover,* an 8-day celebration of the exodus from Egypt during which no unleavened food must be eaten.
- *Hannukkah,* Festival of Lights, during which it is traditional to eat foods cooked in oil, such as doughnuts and potato pancakes.

AFRO-CARIBBEANS

This is an ethnic group and not a religion, but some members, particularly older individuals, have beliefs and customs that may affect health-related behaviour. These may include distinct beliefs about blood categorised as being either "good" or "bad". "Bad" blood indicates poor health and may be the result of incorrect eating habits. Some of the practices for keeping blood "good" (healthy eating, taking exercises, home remedies, using laxatives) are positive and should be included in an individualised diabetes plan.

Many Afro-Caribbeans do not appreciate the association between the presence of obesity and the development of type 2 diabetes.

► KEY POINTS

- Depression and anxiety are more common in diabetics than in the general population.

- The interaction between mental health and diabetes can lead to a vicious cycle of worsening diabetic management and mental illness.

- Driving in diabetics is now subject to a range of legal provisions.

- Diabetics should be immunised against influenza and pneumococcal pneumonia.

- Altering working hours can disrupt eating and sleeping patterns in diabetics, and may worsen glycaemic control, particularly if the rotation pattern is rapid.

- Physically demanding work at unexpected times increases the risk of hypoglycaemia. Patients on insulin should consider using one of the newer basal insulins if working shifts.

- Diabetics should carry sufficient and suitably packed supplies of their medication, supplies, testing equipment, and documentation for their trip. If flying, then these should be packed in carry-on luggage, not stowed.

- To avoid hypoglycaemia or marked hyperglycaemia, diabetics should run their blood sugars slightly higher than normal, particularly during long journeys. If travelling across time zones or eating at unpredictable times, then treatment regimens need to be altered.

- Holders of the European Health Insurance Card are entitled to reduced-cost or, sometimes, free essential medical treatment in the European Economic Area and Switzerland, but are still advised to also obtain travel insurance before departure.

- When diabetics become ill, their blood glucose levels are likely to rise, even if there is little or no calorific intake. In some instances, insulin may need to be administered temporarily.

- Since pregnant women with diabetes are at increased risk, the lead in their management should be a specialist obstetric-endocrine clinic in order to achieve best outcomes.

- There are considerable differences and variations in customs, health beliefs, etiquettes and diet among different cultures.

- Irrespective of culture, clear effective communication remains an essential part of the interaction between professional and patient.

- Optimal management of diabetes during both Ramadan and Hajj is possible with careful planning and attention to detail.

CHAPTER 7

THE ORGANISATION AND DELIVERY OF OPTIMAL DIABETES CARE

OVERVIEW

Although the focus of the primary health care team rests with its patients and local community, the delivery of good care is strongly influenced by a larger framework – government policy and the organisation in which the team works. A better understanding of this framework should help teams to organise the best possible delivery of diabetes care within the available resources.

BACKGROUND TO THE CHANGING ORGANISATION OF DIABETES SERVICES

INTRODUCTION

In October 1989, government health departments and patients' organisations from across Europe, under the aegis of the World Health Organization (WHO) and the International Diabetes Federation (IDF), agreed upon a series of recommendations for diabetes care to be implemented. Called the St Vincent Declaration, this set out goals and targets for improved effective care (WHO/IDF 1990, Krans et al 1992). Subsequent initiatives in the UK have built upon this landmark declaration.

GOVERNMENT POLICIES AND NHS CHANGES

Current government health policy aims to deliver an improved quality of service to individual patients and to the whole population (DoH 1998). General practitioners' (GPs) contracts with the National Health Service (NHS) now reflect the government's intention to support and reward improved quality of care in various areas, including diabetes. In order to address the increasing prevalence of the condition, to take account of greater evidence for and availability for effective interventions, and to meet local patient needs, the organisation of diabetes services needs to adopt an integrated approach between primary, secondary and community care.

National Service Frameworks for Diabetes

Government policy to improve the delivery of care throughout the NHS to patients with diabetes is set out in the National Service Framework (NSF) for Diabetes. Its stated aim is to "make the best practice already offered in some places the norm". This NSF was published in two stages:

- The first stage, published in 2001, listed 12 "standards" that define the areas of care that will need to be delivered (see Appendix 2), of which eight are relevant to type 2 diabetes management in primary care (DoH 2002). Text in this book that is specific to these standards is indicated by a box in the margin in which the numbers of the relevant standards are given.

- The second stage, published in 2003 set out a strategic framework on how the NHS would implement the NSF standards over a 10-year programme (uncosted) (DoH 2003).

Authoritative guidelines

The National Institute of Clinical Excellence (NICE) was established as an independent organisation (although government funded) in 1999 to provide guidance on new and existing technologies and to develop clinical guidelines and audit tools. In April 2005, NICE joined with the Health Development Agency to become the new National Institute for Health and Clinical Excellence (still known as NICE). NICE has published technology appraisals on medication (glitazones, long-acting insulin analogues), delivery systems (insulin pump therapy) and patient education models.

The National Clinical Guideline for type 2 diabetes consists of six inter-related guidelines, developed by a multi-professional, multi-agency collaboration with the support of NICE. These guidelines (with regular updating) aim to provide clinical practice recommendations (with the supporting evidence) for health-care professionals in the following key areas:

- *Foot care* (Hutchinson et al 2000, McIntosh et al 2003).
- *Retinopathy* (NICE 2002a, Hutchinson et al 2001).
- *Renal care* (NICE 2002b, McIntosh et al 2002c). However, this is being superseded by the NSF for chronic kidney disease, part 2 published in 2005 (DH Renal NSF Team 2005).
- *Lipids management* (McIntosh et al 2002a), but now superseded by 2005 guidance from the Joint British Societies, which includes all relevant cardiovascular risk factors (Wood et al 2005) and the 2006 NICE technology appraisal on statins (NICE 2006).
- *Blood pressure management* (Hutchinson et al 2002). These were superseded by separate guidelines from NICE (North of England Hypertension Guideline Development Group 2004) and the British Hypertension Society (Williams et al 2004), updated by a single NICE/BHS guideline in 2006 (NICE 2006a).
- *Blood glucose management* (NICE 2002c, McIntosh et al 2002b).

It is arguable that NICE guidance has not always been set out clearly and that some recommendations are inconsistent with its own stated targets, other current authoritative guidance and the results of research. Professionals need to consider this information, but should be prepared to exercise their best clinical judgement to act in the patient's best interests.

Other authoritative guidelines for the management of diabetes are now readily available from:

- The American Diabetes Association (ADA) publishes comprehensive and referenced clinical practice recommendations, updated annually and available on its website (ADA 2007).
- The Scottish Intercollegiate Guidelines Network (SIGN) published its own excellent authoritative guidelines in 2001, reviewed in 2005 (SIGN 2005).

New General Medical Services (GMS) contract

Since the implementation of the new GMS contract (between an individual general practice and its primary care trust) in 2004, some of general practitioners' annual income is "performance related": derived from practices achieving points in the Quality and Outcomes Framework (QOF), which covers a range of clinical, organisational and "patient experience" indicators. The contents and payment stages of the QOF are reviewed and revised on a 2-yearly cycle. For the 2006–2008 cycle, Appendix 3 lists and describes the indicators that are relevant to the delivery of care to diabetics. These are not only the disease-specific indicators, but are also relevant to other clinical and organisational areas.

Performance data from the first year (2004–2005) of QOF showed that, for diabetes, practices across the country achieved, on average with some variations, about 94% of the maximum points available (Khunti 2006, National Diabetes Support Team 2006b).

The diabetes team

Some GPs can also become a GP with a special interest (GPwSI) in diabetes, following suitable approved training. GPsWIs are expected not only to provide higher-quality disease management, but also to act as "clinical leads", whose roles may include monitoring the implementation of NSF guidelines, coordinating local service developments, and linking with secondary and community care.

The importance of other team members in delivering care must not be forgotten. The Primary Care Diabetes Society was created to represent GPs, GPwSIs, practice nurses and clinical assistants who are involved with diabetes. Practice nurses often take a leading role. Some have become nurse practitioners and have taken a supplementary nurse-prescribing course to allow them to make changes to treatments within the context of practice protocols. Primary care diabetes specialist nurses (DSNs), based in the community and funded by PCTs, have advanced skills to support and deliver care across the community.

NHS reorganisation and policy documents

The NHS continues to undergo changes in its organisation. Many of these changes affect how diabetes care is delivered. Government policy has been to reform the delivery of care in the community, particularly with the significant injection of funding into the NHS. A series of policy documents (available on the DoH website) have been published that outline the direction of this reform process. Among these are the new White Paper "Your Health, Your Care, Your Say: a new direction for community services" published in 2006, covering all aspects of the care people need in the community and their own homes (DoH 2006).

The introduction of practice-based commissioning (PBC) may alter radically in some districts the delivery of diabetes care: although quality assurance remains central, implementation of cost management may result in care and resources being shifted from secondary care into the community, possibly into new "frameworks" (National Diabetes Support Team 2006c). Bearing in mind the high proportion of QOF points achieved, practices will probably continue to manage most of their diabetics, but delivery of care for more "complex" individuals or problems may change.

Evaluation of service delivery of diabetes care

The aim of the Healthcare Commission is to promote improvement in the quality of health care and public health in England and Wales. The Commission is committed to annual assessments of the performance of NHS organisations, including components of the diabetes services. A fact sheet summarises this activity (National Diabetes Support Team 2006a).

Patient experience

As part of the QOF, practices are now expected to undertake an annual patient survey, using one of two approved tools (Improving Practice Questionnaire [IPQ], online at *www.cfep.co.uk*, or General Practice Assessment Questionnaire [GPAQ], online at *http://www.gpaq.info/*), reflect upon it and produce an action plan.

AIMS

The delivery of high-quality care to type 2 diabetic patients in primary care requires that their needs are identified clearly and correctly, and that the available resources are used optimally to address these needs. Better outcomes are more likely to result if the delivery of care respects and complements the goals chosen by the patient. Patients should be regarded as the main managers of their disease. Diabetics who understand their disease are more likely to have similar aims to those of a caring professional. Table 7.1 summarises a professional's perspective of suitable aims for the care of individual patients with diabetes.

NSF ◄
3
4
10
11
12

COMPONENTS OF OPTIMAL ORGANISATION WITHIN PRIMARY CARE

Effective delivery of care to diabetics has relied traditionally upon the three Rs of chronic disease management: **R**egistration, **R**ecall and regular **R**eview. "Multifaceted" interventions (such as individualised goal-setting with patients and suitable education) improve the performance of both the practitioners and the organisation, with better outcome measurements of such parameters as blood pressure and glycated haemoglobin (Olivarus et al 2001, Renders et al 2001). A successful "recipe" for diabetes care needs to contain the appropriate "ingredients":

ACTIVE PARTICIPATION OF DIABETIC PATIENTS IN THEIR CARE

NSF ◄
3

If professionals respect their patients' autonomy, then patients are more likely to be able to act as the main managers of their chronic disease.

Attention to the following guiding principles should enhance this autonomy:

QOF
PE2
PE3
PE4

- Type 2 diabetes is a progressive disease that requires regular and staged changes in therapy. Patients must not be made to feel guilty or at fault when these changes occur.
- Treatment plans should be "negotiated" and attempt to incorporate the patient's own chosen goals. Other issues in a patient's life may affect the priority given to these diabetes-related goals.

TABLE 7.1 Suggested aims for diabetes care

*Ensure the earliest possible **detection** of the disease*

***Abolish symptoms** of the disease*

Achieve **optimal blood glucose control**, avoiding extremes of hypoglycaemia and hyperglycaemia

***Prevent** or delay, and provide early treatment of diabetes complications*

Minimise the **risk** and impact **of cardiovascular disease**

Enable patients to play the fullest possible role in the management of their disease, by providing suitable education and psychological support, **maximising self-reliance**

- Interventions should aim to promote and maintain improved self-care behaviour and to maximise freedom and flexibility in the patient's life.
- Where possible, patients should be encouraged to adjust their treatment and be supported in this. Patients will need to know the actual values and the significance of any tests. This requires the professional to identify and address each patient's educational needs. If patients are allowed to make decisions, then they should be allowed, without stigmatisation, to make mistakes from which each patient and the professional can learn.
- The professional should aim to earn and maintain each patient's respect. Solid evidence, where available, should support any guidance given.
- A balance needs to be struck between keeping things as simple as possible and recognising that diabetes is not a simple disease.
- Patients have the right to make choices that may ultimately cause them harm.

PRIMARY HEALTH-CARE TEAM PERSONNEL

The delivery of diabetes care is a "team effort", with the different members of the primary health-care team each playing an important role. In most practices, GPs and practice nurses will deliver most of the first-line clinical care with administrative and/or reception staff providing the organisational back-up. However, an increasing number of practices have employed or access other professionals:

- Podiatrists
- Dieticians
- Psychologists
- Pharmacists, particularly for medicines management, which may reduce HbA1c results (Choe et al 2005)
- Informatics staff
- Opticians
- Diabetes specialist nurses.

The following points may inform how members of the primary health-care team can deliver diabetes care more effectively:

- The *active leadership* of a GP or a practice nurse with a particular interest in diabetes is likely to provide the necessary driving force within the team.
- Members of the practice involved in any activity require *sufficient and updated knowledge and skills* to undertake these tasks. Training needs should be identified by appraisals, audit, questionnaires and patient feedback. Training may be obtained from a variety of sources, such as attendance at specific courses, observation of specialist colleagues or clinics, distance learning, self-directed reading, or in-house. Current educational practice suggests all team members should have a personal learning plan.
- *Non-medical members* of the team play an important role. With adequate training and safeguards, nurses should be able to prescribe changes in therapy according to an agreed protocol; this enables a prompt and more effective response to problems and a greater likelihood that the individual patient's goals will be achieved.
- *Good working relationships* with others involved in diabetes care outside the practice, both in health and in other services (e.g. social), will facilitate each patient's access to and a more seamless movement between the available agencies that best address each particular need.
- All team members should be *committed to ensuring equitable access and care* to patients of all ethnic and cultural backgrounds.

Chapter 6 of the Diabetes NSF *Delivery Strategy* (DoH 2002) outlines issues that relate to workforce planning and development. Although directed more at a district level, the document and its references may be relevant to how individual practices might manage their own personnel.

ADMINISTRATIVE STRUCTURES AND PROCESSES

NSF ◄
4

The following should enhance the delivery of quality diabetes care in practices:

QOF ◄
DM19

1. An accurate up-to-date *diabetic register* for recall, management and audit, with a named person responsible for maintaining it. All team members should notify the register when made aware of a newly diagnosed or registered diabetic. Practices should also consider setting up a parallel register of those at higher risk of developing diabetes (in particular those with IGT), for recall to be screened regularly.
2. An *evidenced-based protocol* to cover all the key areas of diabetes care within the practice. As a minimum, the protocol needs to provide the framework and details of how the practice will attempt to achieve the maximum points for the various indicators found in the QOF of the GMS contract. The evidence for each component of the protocol may come from various authoritative sources: the latest NICE guidelines and technology appraisals, Diabetes UK recommendations (including Diabetes UK 2000), guidelines from the Joint British Societies (Wood et al 2005)

and the British Hypertension Society, ADA (ADA 2007), and SIGN (SIGN 2001). There may be other sources for ideas, such as locally produced guidelines. Regular audit and reviews of medical literature should enable the protocol to be revised in accordance with best current practice.

3. An effective *call and recall system* should be in place. Administrative and clinical members need to agree upon the precise protocol (including standard recall letters) for contacting diabetic patients when and after their periodic review is due.

4. *Contact details* (telephone and fax numbers, and e-mail addresses) *of and good working relationships with outside professionals*, such as diabetes specialist nurses, podiatrists and hospital diabetic, renal and eye clinics.

5. The *framework for undertaking* both full and interim *diabetes reviews* should be agreed. Adequate time must be set aside within the framework to carry out properly the activities set out in the diabetic protocol. Mini-clinics are regular sessions set aside for diabetes care by the primary health-care team, with regular participation from other professionals. If blood tests are taken prior to the mini-clinic, relevant information is available at the time of review. Figure 7.1 shows a possible model of how patients might "travel" through a practice framework for diabetes care.

6. Practices may wish to look imaginatively at *alternatives to the standard appointment* in the surgery or a home visit, particularly in lifestyle interventions. Examples include telephone prompting, group sessions, electronic and written educational packages, and the involvement of professionals from outside the primary health-care team.

7. Outside of planned reviews, diabetics should have *adequate access* to diabetes care at other times. Nonwhite ethnicity and socio-economic deprivation may affect both needs and access to care. Women with diabetes reported greater difficulties than men in accessing suitable care in practice (Hippisley-Cox et al 2006).

8. The practice should be capable of and willing to undertake regular quality control and *audit,* and to implement changes.

9. The practice must ensure that *adequate resources* are available for the relevant team members to carry out the entire range of tasks required to provide a high-quality service, without detriment to other professional activities.

INFORMATION MANAGEMENT

Optimal information management is an essential ingredient in achieving improved quality in any area of health care. Strategic planning in this area needs to look at what is recorded and how information is handled. Practices may wish to refer to the DoH's documents *Diabetes Information Strategy* (DoH Diabetes Information Strategy 2003) and *Information for Health* (NHS Executive 1998).

Manual records now have only an archive role. The National Programme for Information Technology (NPfIT) is an ambitious national programme to develop an IT

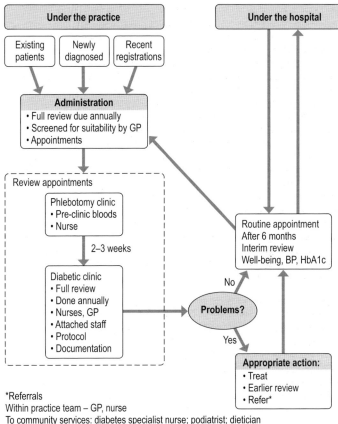

Fig. 7.1 Pathway of patients through a practice diabetes care framework

system in the NHS. Among its elements that will be relevant to the delivery of care to patients with diabetes are patient records (National Care Records Service), electronic transfer of prescriptions (Electronic Prescription Service) and referrals (Choose & Book). The aims are ambitious, but implementation may prove problematic and the track record of national government-funded IT programmes has been poor.

Content

The data recorded by each practice are determined by clinical, administrative and medico-legal requirements. Any data recorded must have a clear purpose and should not be only "for information's sake". QOF indicators and the components of the periodic review could provide the basis for the data that practices wish to record. Precise definitions of all recorded data need to be agreed and understood by all users. All current UK electronic systems use Clinical Terms, known as Read Codes, which are produced and maintained by the NHS Information Authority (NHSIA online). Read Codes for the QOF have been agreed and the relevant documents available from the General Practice Committee of the BMA (West Midlands Local Medical Committee online). Where multiple codes are available for single or similar terms, practices should agree a unique code for each item of data to be recorded and ensure that it will be counted in the QOF.

System design

The design of any information system must address:

- Recording of data
- Data storage
- Data retrieval.

Recording of data

Data recording needs to be accurate, efficient and facilitate retrieval. Diabetic data are best recorded onto agreed specific templates, which facilitate data collection and accessibility. With the new GMS contract, the accredited GP software companies now incorporate templates for recording data required to assess performance of the indicators in the QOF. Protocols need to be developed as to who actually enters data onto the computer. It is also necessary to devise a practical and accurate system for recording data produced from outside the practice (e.g. hospital clinics) onto the practice database.

Data storage

Electronic records should be stored automatically on the practice computer's hard drive, but regular back-up stored off site is required in the event of crashes or other disasters.

Many patients and professionals support the creation of patient-held records to facilitate patient self-management and communication between different centres of care. However, it is necessary that all involved professionals have continuous access to the data. Electronic systems should minimise the time and effort devoted to duplicate data entry onto the practice database.

Data retrieval

It is essential that all relevant data are readily available both to the patient and to the involved health-care professional. With the increasing use of audit for administrative (e.g. contracts) and clinical purposes, the speed and accuracy of retrieving data for analysis on an electronic system is seen to far outweigh the initial extra effort of data entry. The storage and retrieval of patient data must respect all the relevant legal requirements, in particular the Data Protection Acts. This is a minefield, and any practice is well advised to have in place clear policies and suitable training for all involved staff.

PHYSICAL PREMISES AND EQUIPMENT

Practices that carry out diabetes care have a need for the following (which may have "resource implications"):

- *Adequate space*: including access to a darkened room for retinal screening, by whatever method (ophthalmoscope, slit-lamp or retinal camera).
- *For clinical examination:* a sphygmomanometer (with standard and large cuffs), an ophthalmoscope, mydriatic drops (tropicamide 0.5% and 1.0%), tape measure, weighing scales, height measure, cotton wool, patella hammer, tuning fork (128 Hz), sterile needles, 10 g (5.07) monofilaments or Neurotips (if available), Snellen chart for visual acuity hung at the correct distance, pinhole for correction of refractive errors.
- *For testing*: laboratory sample equipment (tourniquet, needles, syringes, blood and urine sample bottles, sharps container, disposable gloves and swabs), urine test strips (for protein, glucose and ketones), blood glucose meter and appropriate test strips (ensure proper quality control) and finger-pricking devices.
- *For therapeutic indications*: glucose for OGTT, and access to insulin and glucagon.
- *For recording and management*: a networked computer terminal with access to a printer for prescriptions and health education literature.
- *For reference:* BNF, BMI chart, and important telephone numbers.

PATIENT INFORMATION AND SUPPORT

A wide range of information is currently available in several formats. Effective health education should ensure that patients have ready access to appropriate up-to-date information as a means of "empowering" them to better self-manage their condition.
Patient information may include:

- *Educational materials* (leaflets, posters and videos) in appropriate languages for nonEnglish-speaking patients, if required.
- *Information on local services*, including optician, dietician, podiatrist and social services.
- *Lists of useful websites* for patients with access to the internet. Some excellent patient information websites include:
  - Diabetes UK: (*www.diabetes.org.uk*)
  - the NHS: *www.patient.co.uk* – then enter "diabetes mellitus" in search
  - Clinical Evidence: *http://www.besttreatments.co.uk/btuk/conditions/6537.jsp*
  - The National Institutes of Health (in the USA): *http://health.nih.gov/result. asp/187.*

Patients and their families may also benefit from support beyond that offered by their professionals. Patients (and families) who join Diabetes UK gain access to a confidential helpline, useful publications and various insurance and financial "products"; there are also better opportunities to meet other people with diabetes.

As discussed above in this section, ready access to professional help (outside the periodic review) is essential for managing various medical problems. During out of hours, patients may find it useful to telephone NHS Direct on 0845 46 47.

DELIVERING HIGH-QUALITY CARE TO OLDER PATIENTS WITH TYPE 2 DIABETES

Type 2 diabetes in the elderly may pose both clinical and logistical problems. With the growing number of older individuals, the prevalence of older diabetics will also increase significantly. Older diabetics are also more likely to request out-of-hours consultations and to need acute hospital admission (Tattersall & Page 1998).

Guidelines for the care of older diabetics have been published by the American Geriatric Society (Brown et al 2003) and the European Diabetes Working Party for Older People (Sinclair et al 2006). The latter suggests that "areas of clinical importance and targets for concerted action" in older diabetics should include:

- functional and vascular risk assessment
- detection of cognitive impairment and depression
- management of specific major complications
- ethical and moral aspects of treatment

  and

- "Care Home" diabetes.

OLDER POPULATION

The prevalence of diabetes is higher in an older than in a younger population. Both clinically and functionally older diabetics are not a homogeneous population. Many will have a variety of co-existing morbidities and more complex medication regimens (with the attendant risks of polypharmacy) than younger people. Older diabetics are more likely to have cognitive impairment and/or depression, and to be more prone to falls, incontinence and chronic pain.

Due to the increasing prevalence of diabetes with increasing age and to frequent asymptomatic presentation, clinicians need to have a lower threshold for considering the diagnosis and arranging appropriate screening. Although the OGTT is the ideal diagnostic test, a fasting plasma glucose may be a more feasible test, and an HbA1c greater than 7.5% may be useful if the individual is frail, demented or confined to a residential home (Greci et al 2003).

ASSESSMENTS

In addition to assessing the components of the periodic review, older patients with diabetes may benefit from an evaluation of:

- *Global/physical function*, such as looking at basic activities of daily living (ADL) (Katz et al 1963)
- *Cognitive function*, such as assessing memory and orientation using the Mini Mental State Examination score (MMSE) (Folstein et al 1975)
- *Nutritional status*, using some agreed checklist or inventory.

TREATMENT AIMS

It remains important that, irrespective of age, all patients are treated with respect and according to their needs, and with full information and access to all appropriate services. There is less evidence for the benefits of tight glycaemic control, blood pressure, and lipid control in individuals over 65 years of age than for the younger population. The recommended targets may need to be reviewed, particularly if there are present other co-morbidities and/or high dependency and/or advanced dementia.

Although glycaemic control is important in older diabetics, the greatest reduction in morbidity and mortality may result from some improvement in all modifiable cardiovascular risk factors. Treating hypertension in the elderly has been shown to be beneficial. There is less evidence for benefits of lipid modification and aspirin therapy; nevertheless, since all diabetics (especially the elderly) are at increased risk for developing CVD, these interventions are worth considering, unless contraindicated or in the very frail with limited life expectancy. Older diabetics who "are active, cognitively intact, and willing to undertake the responsibility of self-management should be encouraged to do so and be treated using the stated goals for younger adults with diabetes" (ADA 2007).

The possible reasons for poor concordance with or refusal of treatment include depression, cognitive impairment, loneliness, adverse socio-economic circumstances and the presence of malignancy. The decision to offer an intervention should take into account the likely benefit/risk ratio. In the elderly, limited life expectancy and increased vulnerability to adverse and other effects may alter the calculation. Health education in the elderly remains as important as any age group, but the content and delivery of the educational package may be altered by sensory and/or cognitive impairment, and other physical frailties.

CARE HOMES

With increasing age, individuals are more likely to be house-bound or live in some form of residential or nursing home. The nature and quality of provision of diabetes care within residential care homes is variable. Among the potential or existing problems that may be encountered in these institutions are:

- Increasing numbers of "clients"
- Lack of access to the full range of health-care professionals, including specialists
- Inadequate dietary care and advice
- Lack of education and training plans for staff
- Lack of individualised care plans
- Poor monitoring of quality.

Staff in homes or other carers can feel isolated and, with numerous other demands upon their time, may not invariably monitor diabetic control and other problems optimally. Practices will need to organise the provision of domiciliary diabetes care for some individuals, in collaboration with other professionals, such as diabetes specialist nurses, podiatrists and opticians, and with the carer(s), who may require education and other support from the practice team. It is crucial that the management protocols are appropriate (not too complex or inflexible) and agreed by all those involved. Ideally, one motivated knowledgeable person should take overall responsibility.

THE NEWLY DIAGNOSED PATIENT

ESSENTIAL QUESTIONS TO BE ADDRESSED AT THE INITIAL CONTACT

When the diagnosis of diabetes is made, three questions need to be answered by the clinician by the end of that initial consultation:

1. **Is the patient severely ill?**

   If yes, then an intercurrent illness may also be present in addition to type 2 diabetes, and the patient should be admitted urgently to hospital, irrespective of the blood glucose level.

2. **Can this patient be managed in a primary care setting?**

   Type 2 diabetics, who have treatable complications should be referred promptly to the appropriate specialist department. However, it is likely that the practice team will become involved in the subsequent management of these problems and of the diabetes.

3. **What treatment is required to correct the blood glucose level?**

   Correction of elevated blood glucose begins at diagnosis. Using the "step-up" recommendations outlined in Table 3.3, the initial choice of diet alone, oral hypoglycaemic agents or insulin (if ketonuria is present) is based upon the following:
   - Current blood glucose level
   - Presence or absence of ketones in the urine
   - Presence of hyperglycaemic symptoms, such as polydipsia and polyuria

- Patient's weight
- Patient's general well-being, hepatic and renal function.

IMPORTANT AREAS TO ADDRESS FROM DIAGNOSIS

At or soon after diagnosis, three further areas will require attention:

1. Involving the patient in the self-management of his or her disease
2. Minimising cardiovascular risk

    and

3. Carrying out essential administrative tasks.

INVOLVING THE PATIENT IN SELF-MANAGEMENT

From the first consultation, health-care professionals need to educate patients about their condition, and allow the patients to make informed choices, wherever possible, about their management.

MINIMISING CARDIOVASCULAR RISK

An early assessment of overall vascular risk, followed by interventions to reduce or eliminate treatable risk factors, such as blood pressure, smoking and lipid profile, should be an integral part of the management of type 2 diabetes.

IMMEDIATE ADMINISTRATIVE TASKS

The urgency of addressing these needs depends upon the patient's circumstances and clinical status.

EARLY ASSESSMENT AND MANAGEMENT

The newly diagnosed type 2 patient requires an early full assessment to detect diabetes complications and cardiovascular risk factors, to identify any specific needs and to tailor management to these findings. This can be done either in the next available diabetic clinic session (if held regularly) or over a series of appointments. The components of the full periodic review are the basis of this assessment, which does need to be more comprehensive to establish a baseline. Additional information gathering will be dictated by the clinical situation. The structure of this assessment involves history, examination, investigations and administrative tasks (see Table 7.2), and will form the basis of the patient's management plan. Optimal outcomes

TABLE 7.2 Components of a full assessment of a newly diagnosed patient with type 2 diabetes

History

Symptoms related to hyperglycaemia (i.e. thirst, polyuria, weight loss, tiredness)
Symptoms that may be related to diabetes complications: visual disturbance, angina, foot problems, sensory disturbances, diarrhoea, infections (balanitis, candidiasis) and male impotence
History and treatment of any other conditions
Lifestyle (i.e. smoking, alcohol consumption, exercise, diet, other substance use)
Family history of diabetes and/or vascular disease
Social circumstances (e.g. occupation, others at home, cultural factors, health beliefs)
Mental status (e.g. cognitive function, affect – including any features of depression)

Examination

Height and weight to give BMI (kg/m^2) and/or record waist circumference
Blood pressure: sitting and standing
Feet: sensation, pulses, skin lesions
Eyes: visual acuity, lens, fundus via dilated pupils
Oral examination
Thyroid palpation
Cardiac examination and peripheral pulses
Abdominal examination (e.g. for hepatomegaly and arterial bruits)
Neurological examination (e.g. for neuropathy)

Investigations

Serum biochemistry: urea and electrolytes (including eGFR), liver function
Serum total cholesterol, lipoprotein fractions and triglycerides
Thyroid function tests
Urinary albumin–creatinine ratio (ACR)

Administrative tasks

Add to diabetic and annual influenza immunisation registers
Invite for pneumococcal immunisation if never administered before or for repeat immunisation either if with another immuno-comprising problem (see BNF) or if over 64 years of age and had previous immunisation more than 5 years previously
Sign the FP92A form, available from chemists, for free prescriptions (patients on insulin or an oral hypoglycaemic are eligible). This is sent to the Health Authority, which issues the patient with an exemption certificate
Advise any drivers that they must notify the DVLA in Swansea that they are now a diabetic and document this advice in their notes. Drivers should also be advised to notify their motor insurance company
Recommend joining Diabetes UK, which can advise on various issues
For patients who are started on hypoglycaemic medication, ensure that they always carry instant sugar and a card to indicate that they are diabetic, what treatment they are on and instructions for dealing with hypoglycaemia
Update repeat prescription and medication review data

are more likely if the patient understands and agrees with the aims and methods. The familiar acronym RAPRIO (reassurance, advice, prescription, referral, investigations, observation) provides a useful framework to organise management interventions.

THE PERIODIC REVIEW: WHAT SHOULD IT CONTAIN?

Although each professional encounter with a diabetic patient provides an opportunity to address any current or potential problems related to lifestyle, glycaemic control, cardiovascular risk, diabetes complications or living with the disease, a systematic regular review ensures that no important aspect of diabetes care is overlooked for all recalled patients on a practice's diabetes register.

Deciding what to include in the periodic review needs to take into account the following:

- Components that will contribute to achieving the most important aims of diabetes care for all patients with diabetes: optimising glycaemic control, minimising cardiovascular risk, minimising diabetes complications and enabling the patient to live with and better self-manage his disease.
- What will enable practices to achieve their maximum QOF points?
- What can be delivered effectively using the current resources of the practices, without detriment to other aspects of patient care?

A suggested list of the essential components for a periodic review is given in Table 7.3. Accurate recording of what is measured is essential.

It is essential, if attempting to achieve optimal outcomes for diabetics, that patient-centred care is both delivered by appropriate members of the team and based upon a "structured, protocol-driven, multi-factorial approach" (Marshall & Flyvbjerg 2006). To avoid fragmenting care by focussing upon specific risk factors and/or complications to the exclusion of all relevant components, it is useful to remember the "Alphabet Strategy" (Lee et al 2004):

- **A**dvice (patient education)
- **B**lood pressure reduction
- **C**holesterol (total and LDL-C)
- **D**iabetes control
- **E**ye care
- **F**eet care
- "**G**uardian drugs" for CVD prevention: aspirin (in most), statin (in most), ACE/ARB (in many), unless contraindicated.

REFERRALS OUTSIDE THE PRIMARY HEALTH-CARE TEAM

Although indications and mechanisms of referral to specialists (mainly secondary care) are discussed throughout the previous sections, a quick reference summary

TABLE 7.3 Suggested minimum set of components for the periodic diabetes review

Aim of diabetes care	Component	Relevant QOF indicator(s)	Comments
Optimising glycaemic control	1. Symptoms of hyperglycaemia and/or hypoglycaemia 2. Self-monitoring results 3. Glycosylated haemoglobin	DM5, DM20 & DM7	
Minimising cardiovascular risk	4. Obesity (BMI) 5. Smoking 6. Physical activity 7. Blood pressure 8. Lipids 9. Anti-platelet therapy	DM2, OB1 Smoking 1 & Smoking 2 DM11 & DM12 DM16 & DM17	HDL-C & LDL-C Unless C/I
Minimising diabetes complications	10. Eyes 11. Kidneys 12. Feet 13. Neuropathy 14. Erectile dysfunction (if applicable) 15. Injection sites (if applicable)	DM21 DM13, DM22, DM15, CKD2, CKD3 & CKD4 DM9 & DM10 DM10	Retinal photo eGFR, ACR
Improving quality of life	16. Depression screening 17. Immunisations against influenza and pneumonia	DEP1 & DEP2 DM18	Use PHQ-2 tool
Administration	18. Medication review 19. Date of next review 20. Data entry		

(not exhaustive) is provided in Table 7.4. Patient safety must remain paramount: clinicians should recognise the limits of their own competence and act accordingly.

MEASURING PERFORMANCE: AUDIT

WHAT IS AUDIT?

"Audit is the process of looking critically and systematically at our own professional activities with a view to improving personal/practice performance and the quality and/or

TABLE 7.4 Summary of possible indications for referral to specialist care

Parameter	Indication	Direction of referral	Where discussed
General well-being	"Looks ill" and presence of intercurrent illness	Consider hospital admission (particularly if socially isolated)	Section VII
General advice	Newly diagnosed – needing broad-based educational input	DESMOND project (if available)	Section II
Diet	When type 2 diabetes is diagnosed When insulin is started When other medical problems are present When HbA1c remains persistently raised If the patient fails to achieve or maintain optimal body weight	Dietician	Section II
Glycosylated haemoglobin	Persistently raised, despite step-up medication – for insulin conversion	Local diabetes specialist nurse	Section III
Hyperglycaemia	If "marked" (threshold for concern will vary depending upon other factors) or risk of significant metabolic abnormalities	Contact local diabetes team or consider hospital admission	Section III
Raised blood pressure	Failure to control on standard combinations Target organ damage Likely underlying cause	Hypertension clinic	Section IV
Dyslipidaemia	Failure to achieve targets Problems with medication	Lipid clinic	Section IV

Continued

TABLE 7.4 Summary of possible indications for referral to specialist care—cont'd

Parameter	Indication	Direction of referral	Where discussed
Obesity	Morbid obesity that fails to respond to diet and medication (in a motivated patient)	Obesity clinic (may be candidate for surgery)	Section IV
Eyes	Cataracts affecting visual acuity Hard exudates <1 dd from fovea or macular oedema or unexplained findings or pre-proliferative retinopathy or more advanced (severe) retinopathy New vessels Retinal detachment	Ophthalmologist (degree of urgency varies)	Section V
Nephropathy	Renal function deteriorating in patients with diabetic nephropathy (particularly to CKD Stages 4 or 5) CKD Stage 3 with other co-morbidity	Nephrologist	Section V

Feet	High-risk foot	Local hospital-based specialist diabetes team	Section V
	Suspected peripheral vascular disease	Vascular surgeon	
	Active foot disease	Multidisciplinary foot care team (within 24 hours)	
	Emergency foot problem	Admission for in-patient care	
Neuropathy	Failure to control pain	Pain clinic	Section V
	Nerve compression	Surgeon	
Erectile dysfunction	Psychological issues	Sex therapist	Section V
	No previous erection and/or severe vascular problem and/or if the intervention is beyond the practitioner's competence	Urologist	
	Hormone abnormality	Endocrinologist	
Depression	Severe (either significant risk of self harm or marked effect on physical health)	Psychiatrist	Section VI
Pregnancy	In existing diabetes or with onset of gestational diabetes	Specialist obstetric-endocrine clinic	Section VI

cost effectiveness of patient care" (Fraser 1982). Guidance for undertaking clinical audit has been set out in *Principles for Best Practice in Clinical Audit*, published in March 2002 (NICE QUIDS 2002). Quality Indicators for Diabetes Services (QUIDS) has developed an audit methodology "appropriate for measuring the clinical quality performance of population based (primary and secondary care) routine, continuing diabetes care". The final report commissioned by NICE, Diabetes UK and the NHS Executive Northwest, is now available (NICE CHI 2002) and complements the Diabetes Information Strategy.

STAGES OF CLINICAL AUDIT, AS APPLIED TO DIABETES CARE

The process is divided into five stages, although not all of the steps in each stage are needed in every audit:

1. Prepare for audit
The steps involved include:

- Involve users (staff, patients) in the process.
- Topic selection, influenced by the team's interests and requirements, and by clinical governance considerations (local and NSF). Table 7.5 suggests aspects of diabetes care that may be suitable for audit, alongside the periodic review.
- Define the purpose of the audit ("to improve, to enhance, to ensure or to change").
- Provide the necessary structures so that audit is an integral part of the team's work.
- Identify and provide the skills, people (including training) and resources required.

2. Select criteria
A *criterion* (plural *criteria*) is an explicit statement that defines the element of care that is being measured. "Valid" criteria should be based upon evidence and related to aspects of care important to the team and/or patient. Criteria can be classified into three groups:

1. Structure (what is needed)
2. Process (what is done)
3. Outcome of care (what is to be expected).

Standards are the percentage of events that should comply with the criterion (Baker 1995). If standards are set, they need to be agreed by the team, based upon relevant high-quality research evidence (if available) and realistic (current targets for glycaemic control, lipids and blood pressure are not always attainable). As the aim of the audit is to improve care, standards may be reset just above the predicted level of performance.

3. Measure performance
Planning data collection
The team needs to identify the group of patients to be studied, the time period over which the criteria apply and the type of data analysis to be used, in order to increase precision and ensure the collection of only essential data.

TABLE 7.5 Aspects of diabetes care suitable for audit (Griffin & Kinmouth 1997)

Criteria group	Suitable examples
1. **Structures** (resources required)	*Availability of specific items* (e.g. a large sphygmomanometer cuff, protocol) *Availability of specific facilities* (e.g. dark room for fundoscopy, educational resources, protected time for reviews) *Practice diabetic register*: does the practice's prevalence equal the local estimate? What is the ethnicity of the diabetic population? *Training* for team members
2. **Processes** (actions and decisions taken by practitioners together with users)	*Appointments* – waiting times and default rate *Record* in the notes of checks of parameters for periodic review agreed in the practice protocol *Uptake* of influenza and pneumonia vaccination in type 2 patients *Information* given to patients as part of their education
3. **Outcomes** (measures of the physical or behavioural response to an intervention, reported health status or level of knowledge and satisfaction); some of these can be used as performance indicators to measure progress in: • medication and diet • implementing the NSF • meeting the St. Vincent Task Force objectives	*Results of parameters* checked *Complications*, e.g. registrable blindness, renal failure, lower limb amputations *Significant events* (e.g. referrals, emergency hospital admissions, deaths, incidence of myocardial infarction) *Levels of patient knowledge* about self-monitoring *Days off work* *Quality of life*

Identifying the study population

An accurate, up-to-date diabetic register enables the whole relevant population to be studied.

Handling data

Data need to be recorded accurately, with the coding agreed and in the most retrievable form. The existing information system may be adequate to provide the necessary data. It is valuable to check a sample of records, looking at free text and file attachments (e.g. outpatient attendances, opticians' reports) to assess the completeness of data capture. The protocol for data extraction should be clear and agreed.

Analysing data
Data analysis can range from a simple calculation of percentages to more sophisticated statistical techniques. Simple methods are usually preferable.

Presenting findings
The findings should be presented clearly, with appropriate use of graphs and tables. It is common for the standard of performance against the agreed criteria to be worse than expected or hoped for. The team then needs to analyse the reason(s) for this shortfall, and so to improve the standard of performance in the future.

Ethical and legal implications
Data collection may have ethical and legal implications, especially in respect of confidentiality. The regulations set out in the Data Protection Act 1998 (HMSO 1997) must be followed. Professional bodies, such as the General Medical Council (General Medical Council 2000) and the Nursing and Midwifery Council, have issued relevant guidance.

4. Make improvements

Practices should have in place the structure to support efforts to make improvements, including professional development. Improved future performance will be more likely if the action plan:

- Is negotiated and agreed within the practice, a process in which barriers to change need to be identified and tackled
- Involves teamwork and ownership of the planned changes

  and

- Is specific, with clearly defined tasks and accountability for each team member.

  Action plans should include a timetable for the next data collection and revised standards for performance against each criterion.

5. Sustain improvement

Sustaining improvement is an extension of the structures and processes by which improvements are made. Lessons learned from audits, critical events and high-quality evidence-based guidance need to be incorporated into routine care. Regular learning activities that improve the knowledge and skills of the team in a focussed way, based upon individual and team needs, should be one of a practice's priorities.

▶ KEY POINTS

- Diabetics are the main managers of their chronic disease, with professionals acting as both guide and coach.
- The aims of diabetes care for each individual should be to:
  - ensure the earliest possible detection of the disease
  - abolish symptoms of the disease
  - achieve optimal blood glucose control, to avoid hypoglycaemia
  - prevent and provide early treatment of any potential complications
  - reduce the risk and impact of cardiovascular disease

and

  - enable patients to play the fullest possible role in the management of their disease, by providing suitable education and psychological support.
- The components of optimal organisation include:
  - active participation of diabetic patients in their own care
  - access to committed trained professionals with a suitable range of skills
  - effective administrative structures and processes
  - optimal information management
  - adequate physical premises and equipment
  - access to suitable information for patients and professionals.
- At diagnosis the answers to the following determine the immediate subsequent management:
  1. Is the patient severely ill?
  2. Can this patient be managed in primary care?
  3. What treatment is required to correct blood glucose?
- The management of older type 2 diabetics poses both clinical and logistical challenges.
- The components of the periodic review need to address each of the aims of diabetes care and to handle administrative requirements that include data entry, follow-up and recall.
- Audit can improve care if undertaken in a systematic way with sensible recommendations for change. Audit can look at structures, processes and outcomes.

FORMULARY OF MEDICATION AVAILABLE IN THE UNITED KINGDOM

Further details are found in the latest editions of the British National Formulary (BNF) and the Monthly Index of Medical Specialties (MIMS). The authors have based the cost calculations on data from the *October* 2007 issues of the Drug Tariff (for generic drugs) and MIMS (for proprietary drugs). The costs are to the NHS, excluding VAT, and are subject to change.

SMOKING CESSATION PRODUCTS

Generic name	Proprietary name(s)	Daily dose range	NHS cost for 28 days(£)
Bupropion	Zyban	150 mg for 6 days; then 150 mg twice daily	37.19
Nicotine	Nicorette Nicotinell NiQuitin CQ	Depends upon preparation	Various
Varenicline	Champix	initially 500 micrograms once daily for 3 days, increased to 500 micrograms twice daily for 4 days, then 1 mg twice daily for 11 weeks (reduce to 500 micrograms twice daily if not tolerated)	54.60

ANTI-OBESITY DRUGS

Generic name	Proprietary name(s)	Daily dose range	NHS cost for 28 days (£)	Comments (see NICE guidance)
Orlistat	Xenical	360 mg in 3 doses after meals	33.58	Lipase inhibitor, reducing dietary fat absorption
Sibutramine	Reductil	10 to 15 mg in 1 dose	36.90–43.65	Centrally acting appetite suppressant, inhibiting re-uptake of norepinephrine (noradrenaline) and serotonin
Rimonabant	Acomplia	20 mg daily before breakfast	44.00	Selective cannabinoid-1 receptor blocker

BLOOD-PRESSURE-LOWERING DRUGS

Angiotensin converting enzyme (ACE) inhibitors

Generic name	Proprietary name(s)	Daily dose range	NHS cost for 28 days (£)
Captopril	Capoten	12.5 mg in 2 doses to 150 mg in 3 doses	0.36–2.01 (generic) 0.84–27.11 (proprietary)
Cilazapril	Vasace	0.5–5 mg	3.65–13.28
Enalapril maleate	Innovace	2.5–40 mg in 1 to 2 doses	0.37–1.32 (generic) 5.35–25.02 (proprietary)
Fosinopril	Staril	10–40 mg	3.00–7.94 (generic) 11.20–24.18 (proprietary)
Imidapril hydrochloride	Tanatril	2.5–20 mg	3.39–9.20
Lisinopril	Carace Zestril	2.5–80 mg	0.43–5.36 (generic) 6.26–47.56 (proprietary)
Moexipril hydrochloride	Perdix	3.75–30 mg	3.78–17.40
Perindopril	Coversyl	2–8 mg	11.36 (all strengths)
Quinapril	Accupro	2.5–80 mg in 1–2 doses	0.65–6.16 (generic) 4.30–19.50 (proprietary)
Ramipril	Tritace	1.25–10 mg	0.60–1.37 (generic – capsules) 5.30–14.24 (proprietary)
Trandolapril	Gopten Odrik	0.5–4 mg	1.40–11.64

ANGIOTENSIN II RECEPTOR ANTAGONISTS (ARB)

Generic name	Proprietary name(s)	Daily dose range	NHS cost for 28 days (£)
Candesartan cilexetil	Amias	8–32 mg	9.89–16.13
Eprosartan	Teveten	300–800 mg	11.63–31.54
Irbesartan	Aprovel	75–300 mg	10.29–16.91
Losartan potassium	Cozaar	25–100 mg	16.18 (all strengths)
Olmesartan medoxomil	Olmetec	10–40 mg	10.95–17.50
Telmisartan	Micardis	20–80 mg	11.34–14.18
Valsartan	Diovan	40–160 mg	16.44–21.66

RENIN INHIBITOR

Generic name	Proprietary name	Daily dose range	NHS cost for 28 days (£)
Aliskiren	Rasilezx	150 to 300mg once daily	19.80–23.80

BETA BLOCKERS

Generic name	Proprietary name(s)	Daily dose range	NHS cost for 28 days (£)	Comments
Acebutolol	Sectral	400–800 mg in 2 doses	19.18–37.24	Cardioselective (relatively) ISA
Atenolol	Tenormin	50 mg	0.29 (generic) 5.11 (proprietary)	Cardioselective Water-soluble
Bisoprolol fumarate	Cardicor, Emcor, Monocor	5–20 mg	2.31–1.60 (generic-higher dose is cheaper) 11.30–25.36 (proprietary)	Cardioselective
Carvedilol	Eucardic	12.5–50 mg	1.57–4.56 (generic) 9.35–23.36 (proprietary)	Arteriolar vasodilator
Celiprolol hydrochloride	Celectol	200–400 mg	8.63–53.78 (generic) 20.63–41.26 (proprietary)	Water-soluble, ISA, arteriolar vasodilator
Labetalol hydrochloride	Trandate	100–800 mg in 2 doses	3.79–26.36 (generic) 3.79–39.94 (proprietary)	Arteriolar vasodilator
Metoprolol tartrate	Betaloc, Lopresor	100–200 mg in 1–2 doses	1.57–2.60 (generic) 2.57–6.68 (proprietary)	Cardioselective
Nadolol	Corgard	80–240 mg	5.20–15.60	Water-soluble
Nebivolol	Nebilet	2.5–5 mg	4.62–9.23	Cardioselective, arteriolar vasodilator
Oxprenolol hydrochloride	Trasicor	80–320 mg in 2–3 doses	3.73–12.40	ISA
Pindolol	Visken	10–45 mg in 2–3 doses	5.85–26.37	ISA
Propranolol	Beta -Prograne, Inderal LA	160–320 mg in 2 doses	2.14–4.03 (generic) 6.36–13.34 (proprietary)	
Timolol maleate	Betim	5–60 mg in 2 doses	0.97–11.65	

CALCIUM CHANNEL BLOCKERS (CCB)

Generic name	Proprietary name(s)	Daily dose range	NHS cost for 28 days (£)	Comments
Amlodipine besilate	Istin	5–10 mg	1.43–1.17 (generic-higher dose is cheaper) 13.04–19.47 (proprietary)	
Diltiazem hydrochloride	Adizem-XL Angitil-SR or XL Calcicard-CR Dilcardia-SR Dilzem Slozem Tildiem Viazem Zemtard	180–360 mg	Many prices (see latest MIMS)	BNF recommends brand prescribing for longer-acting formulations
Felodipine	Plendil, Cardioplen XL	2.5–20 mg	6.70–12.02	
Isradipine	Prescal	2.5–10 mg in 2 doses	8.27–33.08	
Lacidipine	Motens	2–6 mg	9.51–23.74	
Lercanidipine hydrochloride	Zanadip	10–20 mg	5.80–11.00	
Nicardipine hydrochloride	Cardene Cardene SR	60–120 mg in 3 doses (2 doses if sustained release)	10.21–22.42 (sustained-release) 11.27–22.53 (normal capsules)	
Nifedipine	Adalat Adipine MR Cardilate MR Coracten Fortipine LA Tensipine MR	20–80 mg in 1–2 doses	3.99–17.68 (many prices-see latest MIMS)	Only sustained-release preparations are suitable for hypertension
Nisoldipine	Syscor MR	10–40 mg daily	8.77–35.08	
Verapamil hydrochloride	Cordilox Securon Univer	240–480 mg in 2–3 doses	1.91–23.39 (generic) 5.89–17.26 (proprietary)	

THIAZIDE AND THIAZIDE-LIKE DIURETICS

Generic name	Proprietary name(s)	Daily dose range	NHS cost for 28 days (£)
Bendroflumethiazide	Various	2.5 mg in the morning	0.43 (generic) 1.00–1.18 (proprietary)
Chlortalidone	Hygroton	25–50 mg in the morning	0.82–1.64
Cyclopenthiazide	Navidrex	0.25–0.5 mg in the morning	0.64–1.27
Indapamide	Natrilix	2.5 mg in the morning	1.63 (generic) 4.20 (proprietary)
Metolazone	Metenix 5	5 mg in the morning	5.30
Xipamide	Diurexan	20 mg in the morning	3.89

ALPHA 1 ADRENERGIC BLOCKERS

Generic name	Proprietary name(s)	Daily dose range	NHS cost for 28 days (£)
Doxazosin	Cardura	1–16 mg	0.46–5.96 (generic) 10.56–112.64 (proprietary)
	Cardura XL (modified release)	4–8 mg	6.33–12.67 (modified release)
Indoramin	Baratol	50–200 mg in 2–3 doses	6.00–24.00
Prazosin	Hypovase	1.5 mg in 3 doses to 20 mg	3.77–17.50 (generic) 3.77–32.29 (proprietary)
Terazosin	Hytrin	1–20 mg at bedtime	1.53–23.54 (generic) 2.29–34.28 (proprietary)

ALDOSTERONE ANTAGONIST

Generic name	Proprietary name	Daily dose range	NHS cost for 28 days (£)
Spironolactone	Aldactone	12.5 mg	1.06 (generic) 1.73–4.45 (proprietary)

OTHER ANTIHYPERTENSIVE AGENTS

Generic name	Proprietary names	Daily dose range	NHS cost for 28 days (£)
Clonidine	Catapres	0.15–0.3 mg in 3 doses	1.51–13.04
Hydralazine	Apresoline	50–100 mg in 2 doses	9.45–13.94 (generic) 1.88–3.76 (proprietary)
Methyldopa	Aldomet	500 mg in 2 doses to 3000 mg in 3 doses	6.83–36.93 (generic) 1.75–10.64 (proprietary)
Minoxidil	Loniten	2.5–50 mg	4.14–71.59
Moxonidine	Physiotens	0.2 mg in 1 dose to 0.6 mg in 2 doses	6.71–16.14

COMBINATION ANTIHYPERTENSIVE AGENTS

Proprietary name	Constituents	Description	Daily dose range	NHS cost for 28 days (£)
Accuretic	Quinapril 10 mg/hydrochlorothiazide 12.5 mg	ACE/thiazide diuretic	1–2	11.75–23.50
Acezide	Captopril 50 mg/hydrochlorothiazide 25 mg	ACE/thiazide diuretic	1–2	13.15–26.30
Beta-Adalat	Atenolol 50 mg/nifedipine 20 mg	Beta blocker/ CCB	1–2	10.41–20.82
Capozide	Captopril 50 mg/hydrochlorothiazide 25 mg	ACE/thiazide diuretic	1	7.45
Capozide LS	Captopril 25 mg/hydrochlorothiazide 12.5 mg	ACE/thiazide diuretic	1	10.46
Carace 10 Plus	Lisinopril 10 mg/hydrochlorothiazide 12.5 mg	ACE/thiazide diuretic	1–2	10.51–21.02
Carace 20 Plus	Lisinopril 20 mg/hydrochlorothiazide 12.5 mg	ACE/thiazide diuretic	1–2	11.89–23.78

Continued

COMBINATION ANTIHYPERTENSIVE AGENTS—Cont'd

Proprietary name	Constituents	Description	Daily dose range	NHS cost for 28 days (£)
Co-Diovan	Valsartan 80 or 160 mg/hydrochlorothiazide 12.5 or 25 mg as 80/12.5, 160/12.5 or 160/25	ARB/thiazide diuretic	1	16.44–21.66
Coversyl Plus	Perindopril 4 mg/indapamide 1.25 mg	ACE/diuretic	1 in the morning	14.49
Dyazide	Triamterene 50 mg/hydrochlorothiazide 25 mg	Potassium sparing diuretic/thiazide diuretic	1	0.95
Exforge	Amlodipine 5 or 10 mg + valsartan 80 or 160 mg as 5/80, 5/160 or 10/60	CCB/ARB	1	16.44 (5/80) 21.66 (5/160, 10/60)
Innozide	Enalapril 20 mg/hydrochlorothiazide 12.5 mg	ACE/thiazide diuretic	1–2	13.90–27.80
Kalspare	Chlortalidone 50 mg/triamterene 50 mg	Thiazide diuretic/potassium sparing diuretic	1–2	3.05–6.10
Kalten	Atenolol 50 mg/hydrochlorothiazide 25 mg/amiloride 2.5 mg	ACE/thiazide diuretic/potassium sparing diuretic	1	10.01
Micardis Plus	Telmisartan 40 or 80 mg/hydrochlorothiazide 12.5 mg	ARB/thiazide diuretic	1	11.34–14.18
Moduret 25	Amiloride 2.5 mg/hydrochlorothiazide 25 mg	Potassium sparing diuretic/thiazide diuretic	1–4 in divided doses	0.90–3.60
Moduretic	Amiloride 5 mg/hydrochlorothiazide 50 mg	Potassium sparing diuretic/thiazide diuretic	½–2	1.34–5.28

Olmetec Plus 20/12.5 20/25	Olmesartan 20 mg/hydrochlorothiazide 12.5 mg	ARB/thiazide diuretic	1	12.95
	Olmesartan 20 mg/hydrochlorothiazide 25 mg		1	12.95
Navispare	Cyclopenthiazide 0.25 mg/amiloride 2.5 mg	Thiazide diuretic/ potassium sparing diuretic	1–2	2.70–5.40
Tenif	Atenolol 50 mg/nifedipine 20 mg	Beta blocker/ CCB	1–2	10.63–21.26
Tenoret 50	Atenolol 50 mg/chlortalidone 12.5 mg	Beta blocker/ thiazide diuretic	1	5.70
Tenoretic	Atenolol 100 mg/chlortalidone 25 mg	Beta blocker/ thiazide diuretic	1	8.12
Trasidrex	Oxprenolol 160 mg/cyclopenthiazide 0.25 mg	Beta blocker/ thiazide diuretic	1–2	10.66–21.32
Zestoretic 10	Lisinopril 10 mg/hydrochlorothiazide 12.5 mg	ACE/thiazide diuretic	1–2	13.01–26.02
Zestoretic 20	Lisinopril 20 mg/hydrochlorothiazide 12.5 mg	ACE/thiazide diuretic	1–2	14.72

LIPID-REGULATING DRUGS

Anion-exchange resins

Generic name	Proprietary name(s)	Daily dose range	NHS cost for 28 days (£)
Colestyramine	Questran	1–9 sachets	6.40–57.56 (generic) 9.63–86.64 (sugar free)
Colestipol hydrochloride	Colestid	5–30 g daily in 1 or 2 doses	14.05–84.28

FIBRATES

Generic name	Proprietary name(s)	Daily dose range	NHS cost for 28 days (£)
Bezafibrate	Bezalip,	600 mg in 3 doses	8.74 (generic)
			7.69 (proprietary)
	Bezalip Mono	400 mg in 1 dose	7.55 (Mono)
Ciprofibrate	Modalim	100 mg	17.66
Fenofibrate	Lipantil micro Supralip mono	134–267 mg	14.50–21.75
Gemfibrozil	Lopoid	600 mg twice daily	48.93

STATINS

Generic name	Proprietary name(s)	Daily dose range	NHS cost for 28 days (£)
Atorvastatin	Lipitor	10–80 mg at night	18.03–28.21
Fluvastatin	Lescol	20–80 mg at night	15.26–19.20
Pravastatin sodium	Lipostat	10–40 mg at night	3.40–7.54 (generic) 15.05–27.61 (proprietary)
Rosuvastatin	Crestor	10–40 mg	18.03–29.69
Simvastatin	Zocor	10–80 mg at night	0.34–4.91 (generic) 18.03–29.69 (proprietary)

AZETIDINONES

Generic name	Proprietary name	Daily dose range	NHS cost for 28 days (£)
Ezetimibe	Ezetrol	10 mg	26.31

NICOTINIC ACID GROUP

Generic name	Proprietary name(s)	Daily dose range	NHS cost for 28 days (£)
Acipimox	Olbetam	500–750 mg in divided doses	28.83–43.24
Nicotinic acid	Niaspan (modified release)	1–2 g (modified release)	17.25–29.50

FISH OILS

Generic name	Proprietary name(s)	Daily dose range	NHS cost for 28 days (£)
Omega-3-acid ethyl esters	Omacor	1–4 capsules	13.89–55.56
Omega-3-marine triglycerides	Maxepa	5 capsules twice daily OR 5 ml twice daily	38.19 (both capsules and liquid)

ANTIPLATELET DRUGS

Generic name	Proprietary name(s)	Daily dose range	NHS cost for 28 days (£)

Aspirin:
  dispersible
  enteric coated
		75 mg	0.29 (dispersible)
			0.51 (enteric-coated)

Clopidogrel	Plavix	75 mg	35.31
Dipyridamole modified release	Persantin Retard	200 mg twice daily	7.82

BLOOD GLUCOSE-LOWERING DRUGS

Sulphonylureas

Generic name	Proprietary name(s)	Daily dose range	NHS cost for 28 days (£)	Comments
Tolbutamide		250–2000 mg	0.83–6.64	Short-acting
Gliclazide	Diamicron	40–320 mg (160 mg maximum single dose)	0.33–2.64 (generic) 1.06–8.51 (proprietary)	Excreted in bile

Continued

BLOOD GLUCOSE-LOWERING DRUGS—Cont'd

Sulphonylureas

Generic name	Proprietary name(s)	Daily dose range	NHS cost for 28 days (£)	Comments
Gliclazide MR	Diamicron MR	30–120 mg, in the morning	3.08–12.32	Increments at 2-week intervals
Glipizide	Glibenese Minodiab	2.5–20 mg (15 mg maximum single dose)	1.48–8.16	Before breakfast or lunch
Glimepiride	Amaryl	1–6 mg, at breakfast	3.15–13.83	
Glibenclamide	Daonil Euglycon	2.5–15 mg	0.29–1.02 (generic) 1.73–8.07 (proprietary)	Long-acting

POST-PRANDIAL GLUCOSE REGULATORS

Generic name	Proprietary name(s)	Daily dose range	NHS cost for 28 days (£)	Comments
Repaglinide	Prandin	0.5–16 mg (4 mg maximum single dose) before meals	3.66–29.27	Not recommended in over 75 years
Nateglinide	Starlix	180–540 mg in 3 divided doses	22.71–25.88	Licenced only in combination with metformin

BIGUANIDE

Generic name	Proprietary name	Daily dose range	NHS cost for 28 days (£)
Metformin	Glucophage	500–2000 mg in divided doses	0.34–1.36 (generic) 0.96–3.84 (proprietary)

INCRETIN MIMETICS

Generic name	Proprietary name	Daily dose range	NHS cost for 28 days (£)
GLP-1 analogue Exenatide	Byetta	5 to 10 microgrammes twice daily (injected subcutaneously) before meals	63.69
DPP-4 inhibitor Sitagliptin	Januvia	100mg once daily	33.26

THIAZOLIDINEDIONES

Generic name	Proprietary name(s)	Daily dose range	NHS cost for 28 days (£)	Comments
Pioglitazone	Actos	15–45 mg	24.14–36.96	Monitor LFTs
Rosiglitazone	Avandia	4–8 mg	24.74–50.78	Monitor LFTs; can increase dose after 8 weeks

OTHER BLOOD-GLUCOSE-LOWERING DRUGS

Generic name	Proprietary name	Daily dose range	NHS cost for 28 days (£)
Acarbose	Glucobay	50–600 mg	2.05–21.02

COMBINATION ORAL HYPOGLYCAEMIC AGENTS

Proprietary name	Constituents	Description	Daily dose range	NHS cost for 28 days (£)
Avandamet	2/1000: rosiglitazone 2 mg + metformin 1000 mg	Thiazolidinedione/ biguanide	1 tablet twice daily	27.71
	4/1000: rosiglitazone 4 mg + metformin 1000 mg		1 tablet twice daily	52.45
	2/500: rosglitazone 2 mg + metformin 500 mg		2 tablets twice daily	52.45
Competact	Pioglitazone 15 mg metformin 850 mg	Thiazolidinedione biguanide	1 tablet twice daily with or after food	31.56

IINSULINS

Short-acting

Generic name	Constituents	Proprietary name(s)	NHS cost for 100U (£) depending upon device
Soluble insulin	Bovine, highly purified Porcine, highly purified Human, pyr Human, crb	Hypurin Bovine Neutral Hypurin Porcine Neutral Actrapid Humulin S Insuman Rapid	1.85 1.68 0.75 1.65–1.87 1.56–1.86

Rapid-acting

Generic name	Constituents	Proprietary name(s)	NHS cost for 100U (£) depending upon device
Insulin aspart	Recombinant human insulin analogue	NovoRapid	1.73–2.10
Insulin glulisine	Recombinant human insulin analogue	Apidra	1.73–1.96
Insulin lispro	Recombinant human insulin analogue	Humalog	1.73–1.96

Intermediate- and long-acting

Generic name	Constituents	Proprietary name(s)	NHS cost for 100U (£) depending upon device
Insulin detemir	Recombinant human insulin analogue	Levemir	2.60–2.90 No vials
Insulin glargine	Recombinant human insulin analogue	Lantus	2.60–2.80
Insulin zinc suspension	Bovine, highly purified	Hypurin Bovine Lente	1.85
Isophane insulin	Bovine, highly purified Porcine, highly purified Human sequence	Hypurin Bovine Isophane Hypurin Porcine Isophane Insulatard Humulin I Insuman Basal	1.85 1.68 0.75–1.34 1.65–2.00 1.17–1.86
Protamine zinc insulin		Hypurin Bovine Protamine Zinc	1.85

Biphasic insulins

Generic name	Constituents	Proprietary name(s)	NHS cost for 100U (£) depending upon device
Biphasic insulin aspart	30% insulin aspart, 70% insulin aspart protamine	NovoMix 30	1.96–2.13 No vials
Biphasic insulin lispro	25% insulin lispro, 75% insulin lispro protamine	Humalog Mix25	1.96–2.07 No vials
	50% insulin lispro, 50% insulin lispro protamine	Humalog Mix50	1.96–2.07 No vials
Biphasic isophane insulin	*Highly purified animal:* Porcine, highly purified 30% soluble, 70% isophane	Hypurin Porcine 30/70 mix	1.68
		Pork Mixtard 30 (to be withdrawn December 2007)	0.40
	Human sequence: Human, pyr 10% soluble, 90% isophane	Mixtard 10	1.34 (no vials)
	20% soluble, 80% isophane	Mixtard 20	1.34 (no vials)
	30% soluble, 70% isophane	Mixtard 30	0.75–1.34
	40% soluble, 60% isophane	Mixtard 40	1.34 (no vials)
	50% soluble, 50% isophane	Mixtard 50	1.34 (no vials)
	Human, prb 30% soluble, 70% isophane	Humulin M3	1.65–2.00
	Human, crb 15% soluble, 85% isophane	Insuman Comb 15	1.86 (no vials)
	25% soluble, 75% isophane	Insuman Comb 25	1.17–1.86
	15% soluble, 85% isophane	Insuman Comb 50	1.86 (no vials)

ANALGESIA FOR NEUROPATHY

Tricyclic antidepressants

Generic name	Proprietary name(s)	Daily dose range	NHS cost for 28 days (£)
Amitriptyline		10–75 mg	0.69–2.07
Imipramine		10–75 mg	1.00–2.67
Nortriptyline	Allegron	10–25 mg	3.38–6.73

ANTICONVULSANTS

Generic name	Proprietary name(s)	Daily dose range	NHS cost for 28 days (£)
Gabapentin	Neurontin	900–1800 mg	27.01–89.04
Pregabalin	Lyrica	150–600 mg in 2–3 doses	64.40

ERECTILE DYSFUNCTION

Phosphodiesterase type-5 inhibitors

Generic name	Proprietary name	Dose range (mg)	NHS cost for each treatment
Sildenafil	Viagra	25–100	4.15–5.87
Tadalafil	Cialis	10–20	6.25
Vardenafil	Levitra	10–20	4.15–5.87

Alprostadil

Generic name	Proprietary name	Dose range (mg)	NHS cost for each treatment
Alprostadil	*Intracavernosal injection:* Caverject Viridial Duo	 5–40 10–40	 7.73–21.58 16.55–29.83
	Urethral application MUSE	 125–1000	 10.38–11.56

NATIONAL SERVICE FRAMEWORK STANDARDS FOR DIABETES

Department of Health: National Service Framework for Diabetes Standards (London, HMSO, 2001).

Standard	Where discussed in this book
1. *Prevention:* To reduce the number of people who develop type 2 diabetes	Chapters 1 (prevention) and 2 (dietary advice, physical activity)
2. *Diagnosis:* To ensure that people with diabetes are identified as early as possible	Chapter 1
3. *Empowerment:* To ensure that people with diabetes are empowered to enhance their personal control over the day-to-day management of their diabetes in a way that enables them to experience the best quality of life	Chapters 2 (lifestyle, health education), 3 (glycaemic control) and 6 (aims, organisation, further information)
4. *Clinical Care:* To maximise the quality of life of all people with diabetes and to reduce their risk of developing the long-term complications of diabetes	Chapters 3 (glycaemic control), 4 (cardiovascular risk) and 6 (organisation, recall, periodic review and audit)
5. *Young People With Diabetes:* high-quality care	Mostly type 1 diabetes – not in the scope of this book
6. *Young People With Diabetes:* smooth transition from paediatric to adult services	Not in the scope of this book
7. *Diabetic Emergencies:* To minimise the impact on people with diabetes of the acute complications of diabetes	Chapters 3 (glycaemic control) and 5 (complications)
8. *Hospital Admissions:* Not relevant to primary care	Not in the scope of this book
9. *Diabetes and Pregnancy*	Chapter 6 (pregnancy in type 2 diabetes)
10. *Detection and Management of Long-Term Complications:* All patients with diabetes receive regular surveillance for the long-term complications of diabetes	Chapter 5 (diabetic complications)
11. *Detection and Management of Long-Term Complications:* Implement and monitor agreed protocols of care so that all those who develop complications receive appropriate care	Chapter 7 (organisation of periodic review, audit)
12. *Detection and Management of Long-Term Complications:* All those requiring multi-agency support will receive integrated health and social care	Chapter 5 (complications) and 7 (organisation, periodic review)

NEW GMS CONTRACT INDICATORS (2006–2008)

Online access via: http://www.nhsemployers.org/primary/primary-703.cfm
The pdf is available online: https://www.nhsemployers.org/restricted/
downloads/download.asp?ref=718&hash=50c3d7614917b24303ee6a220679dab3

DIABETES

The new GMS contract has been revised for the cycle 2006–2008.
Compared to the first cycle in 2004–2006:

1. The number of indicators for diabetes has been reduced from 18 to 16
2. Two of the existing indicators have been revised:
   - DM6 upper threshold of HbA1c of 7.4% or less revised in DM20 to 7.5% or less
   - DM14 recording serum creatinine is now DM22, either eGFR or serum creatinine
3. Two of the old indicators have been removed:
   - DM3 and DM4 – smoking
4. Point numbers in two existing indicators have been revised:
   - DM20 (formerly DM6) now 17 points (previously 16)
   - DM12 now 18 points (previously 17)
5. Payment stages have been revised:
   - In all indicators but DM19 (the register), the minimum threshold has been raised from 25% (in 2004–2006) to 40% (2006–2008)
   - In DM7, the maximum payment stage has been increased from 85 to 90%
   - In DM12, the maximum payment stage has been increased from 55 to 60%
   - In DM15, the maximum payment stage has been increased from 70 to 80%
   - In DM17, the maximum payment stage has been increased from 60 to 70%
6. The total number of points has been reduced from 99 to 93.

These indicators are due for review again in 2007–2008, and may change for the following (2008–2010) and subsequent 2-year financial cycles.

Indicator	Points	Payment stages	Where discussed in this book
RECORDS **DM19**: The practice can produce a register of all patients aged 17 years and over with diabetes mellitus, which specifies whether the patient has type 1 or type 2 diabetes	6	Not applicable	Chapters 1 (classification) and 7 (organisation)
ONGOING MANAGEMENT The minimum threshold for all of the below is 40%			
DM2: The percentage of patients with diabetes whose notes record BMI in the previous 12 months	3	40–90%	Chapter 4 (obesity)

DM5: The percentage of diabetic patients who have a record of HbA1c or equivalent in the previous 15 months	3	40–90%	Chapters 3 (HbA1c) and 7 (organisation)
DM20: The percentage of patients with diabetes in whom the last HbA1c is 7.5 or less (or equivalent test/reference range depending on local laboratory) in last 15 months	17	40–50%	Chapters 2 (diet, physical activity), 3 (glycaemic control) and 7 (organisation)
DM7: The percentage of patients with diabetes in whom the last HbA1c is 10 or less (or equivalent test/reference range depending on local laboratory) in last 15 months	11	40–90%	Chapters 2 (diet, physical activity), 3 (glycaemic control) and 7 (organisation)
DM21: The percentage of diabetic patients who have a record of retinal screening in the previous 15 months (identical to previous DM8)	5	40–90%	Chapter 5
DM9: The percentage of patients with diabetes with a record of presence or absence of peripheral pulses in the previous 15 months	3	40–90%	Chapter 5
DM10: The percentage of patients with diabetes with a record of neuropathy testing in the previous 15 months	3	40–90%	Chapter 5
DM11: The percentage of patients with diabetes who have a record of the blood pressure in the past 15 months	3	40–90%	Chapter 4
DM12: The percentage of patients with diabetes in whom the last blood pressure is 145/85 or less	18	40–60%	Chapter 4
DM13: The percentage of patients with diabetes who have a record of micro-albuminuria testing in the previous 15 months (exception reporting for patients with proteinuria)	3	40–90%	Chapter 5
DM22: The percentage of patients with diabetes who have a record of estimated glomerular filtration rate (eGFR) or serum creatinine testing in the previous 15 months	3	40–90%	Chapter 5

Continued

Indicator	Points	Payment stages	Where discussed in this book
DM15: The percentage of patients with diabetes with proteinuria or micro-albuminuria who are treated with ACE inhibitors (or A2 antagonists)	3	40–80%	Chapters 3 (drugs) and 5 (nephropathy)
DM16: The percentage of patients with diabetes who have a record of total cholesterol in the previous 15 months	3	40–90%	Chapter 4
DM17: The percentage of patients with diabetes whose last measured total cholesterol within previous 15 months is 5 mmol/l or less	6	40–70%	Chapter 4
DM18: The percentage of patients with diabetes who have had influenza immunisation in the preceding 1 September to 31 March	3	40–85%	Chapter 6

Although specific diabetes care accounts for 93 points, there are a number of other areas in which delivering high-quality diabetes care can provide further points:

CHRONIC KIDNEY DISEASE

Indicator	Points	Payment stages	Where discussed in this book
ChKD1: The practice can produce a register of patients aged 18 years and over with ChKD (US National Kidney Foundation: Stage 3–5 ChKD)	6	Not applicable	Chapter 5
ChKD2: The percentage of patients on the ChKD register whose notes have a record of blood pressure in the previous 15 months	6	40–90%	Chapter 4
ChKD3: The percentage of patients on the ChKD register in whom the last blood pressure reading, measured in the previous 15 months, is 140/85 or less	11	40–70%	Chapter 4
ChKD4: The percentage of patients on the ChKD register who are treated with an angiotensin converting enzyme inhibitor (ACE-I) or angiotensin receptor blocker (ARB) (unless a contraindication or side effects are recorded)	4	40–80%	Chapter 4

DEPRESSION

Indicator	Points	Payment stages	Where discussed in this book
DEP 1: The percentage of patients with diabetes and/or heart disease for whom case finding for depression has been undertaken on one occasion during the previous 15 months using the two standard screening questions	8	40–90%	Chapter 6
DEP 2: In those patients with a new diagnosis of depression, recorded between the preceding 1 April and 31 March, the percentage of patients who have had an assessment of severity at the outset of treatment using an assessment tool validated for use in primary care	25	40–90%	Chapter 6

OBESITY

Indicator	Points	Where discussed in this book
OB1: The practice can produce a register of patients aged 16 and over with a BMI greater than or equal to 30 in the previous 15 months	8	Chapter 4

SMOKING

Indicator	Points	Payment stages	Where discussed in this book
Smoking 1 (formerly DM3): The percentage of patients with any combination of the following conditions: coronary heart disease, stroke or TIA, hypertension, diabetes, COPD or asthma, whose notes record smoking status in the previous 15 months. Except those who have never smoked where smoking status need only be recorded once since diagnosis	33	40–90%	Chapter 2
Smoking 2 (formerly DM4): The percentage of patients with any or any combination of the following conditions: coronary heart disease, stroke or TIA, hypertension, diabetes, COPD or asthma, who smoke and whose notes record that smoking cessation advice or referral to a specialist service, where available, has been offered within the previous 15 months	35	40–90%	Chapter 2

ORGANISATIONAL DOMAIN

Indicator	Points	Where discussed in this book
RECORDS AND INFORMATION **Record 21:** Ethnic origin is recorded for 100% of new registrations	1	Chapters 5 and 6
EDUCATION AND TRAINING **Education 8**: All practice-employed nurses have personal learning plans, which have been reviewed at an annual appraisal	5	Chapter 6

PATIENT EXPERIENCE DOMAIN

Indicator	Points	Where discussed in this book
PE2 (Patient Surveys 1): The practice will have undertaken an approved patient survey each year	25	Chapter 7
PE3 (Patient Surveys 2): The practice will have undertaken a patient survey each year and, having reflected on the results, will produce an action plan that: 1. Summarises the findings of the survey. 2. Summarises the findings of the previous year's survey 3. Reports on the activities undertaken in the past year to address patient experience issues	20	Chapter 7
PE4 (Patient Surveys 3): The practice will have undertaken a patient survey each year, having reflected on the results, will produce an action plan that: 1. Sets priorities for the next 2 years 2. Describes how the practice will report the findings to patients (for example, posters in the practice, a meeting with a patient practice group or a PCO approved patient representative) 3. Describes the plans for achieving the priorities, including indicating the lead person in the practice 4. Considers the case for collecting additional information on patient experience, for example, through surveys of patients with specific illnesses, or consultation with a patient group	30	Chapter 7

FURTHER READING AND USEFUL CONTACTS

This book is intended as a practical guide. Since diabetes is a rapidly changing field, parts of the text will inevitably become out of date as a result of the publication of new research and yet more official guidelines. Keeping up-to-date involves a regular perusal of suitable internet sites and journals.

EVALUATING NEW INFORMATION

Clinicians need to be able to assess the quality of new information, to identify what is important (may change current practice) and to put aside what is not. This subsection aims to provide an overview of some of the important concepts that may help readers to evaluate new information.

EVIDENCED-BASED MEDICINE: A VERY BRIEF OVERVIEW

Basic concepts

Clinicians need to base their decisions about intervention upon the best available evidence. Practitioners of evidence-based medicine (EBM) argue that effective clinicians should:

1. Ask focused answerable clinical questions in terms of:
   - The patient or problem
   - The intervention
   - The comparison intervention, if appropriate
   - The outcome
2. Search the literature effectively for the best evidence
3. Assess critically the quality of this evidence:
   When evaluating a study, it is useful to ask:
   - Is the population recruited representative of what most GPs see?
   - Can the practice carry out the studied intervention and any associated activities without detriment to the patient or the practice's total portfolio of professional services?
   - Does the presentation of randomised controlled trials (RCTs) conform to the CONSORT guidelines (Chapter 7; Altman et al 2001)?
   - Is the outcome's endpoint both measurable in and relevant to primary care?
   The interpretation of results from some large and important studies, e.g. the UK PDS and HOPE, may not be universally agreed. Even in some important studies that recruited subjects from primary care, the characteristics (often due to exclusions, such as age) and the effect of treatment upon the study subjects may not be representative of the "real" population that present with the same problem to primary care (Chapter 7; Mant et al 2006).
4. Integrate this evidence into a management plan.

The evidence base for recommendations

Many guidance documents now published by authoritative bodies, such as NSF, NICE and SIGN, indicate the type of evidence used to support their recommendations. The classification and definitions of these types of evidence originate from the United States Agency for Health Care Policy and Research. All bodies agree upon the main levels, 1 to 4, but may vary upon how many divisions to include at each level (greater weight of evidence at lowest level):

LEVELS OF EVIDENCE (DEFINITIONS USED BY NICE)

Level	Description
Ia	Evidence from meta-analysis of randomised controlled trials
Ib	Evidence from at least one randomised controlled trial
IIa	Evidence from at least one controlled study without randomisation
IIb	Evidence from at least one other type of quasi-experimental study
III	Evidence from nonexperimental descriptive studies, e.g. comparative studies, correlation studies, case-control studies
IV	Expert opinion (in the absence of any of the above)

The guidance issued by expert bodies often uses a grading scheme for their recommendations:

GRADES OF RECOMMENDATIONS

Grade	Evidence used
A	Directly based upon level I evidence
B	Directly based upon level II evidence, or extrapolated recommendation from level I evidence
C	Directly based upon level III evidence, or extrapolated recommendation from level I or II evidence
D	Directly based upon level IV evidence, or extrapolated recommendation from level I, II or III evidence

EVIDENCE-BASED MEDICINE (EBM) RESOURCES

The two following books are excellent guides for beginners:

1. Sackett DL, Strauss SE, Glaziou P, Richardson WS, Rosenberg W, Haynes RB 2005 Evidence-Based Medicine: How to Practice and Teach EBM, 3rd Edn. Edinburgh: Churchill Livingstone
2. Greenhalgh T 2006 How to read a paper: The basics of evidence based medicine, 3rd Edn. London: BMJ Publishing Group

The following electronic EBM resources may be valuable as a starting point:

1. **Finding answers to questions in EBM** is an excellent Norwegian site in English, based at the University of Bergen, for beginners with useful links: www.uib.no/isf/people/atle/ebm.htm
2. **Netting the Evidence Guide** on: http://www.shef.ac.uk/scharr/ir/netting/

Books
1. Bailey CJ, Krentz AJ 2005 Type 2 Diabetes in Practice, 2nd Edn. London: Royal Society of Medicine Press Limited
2. MacKinnon M 2002 Providing Diabetes Care in General Practice: A Practical Guide for the Primary Care Team, 4th Edn. London: Class Publishing

Journals
1. Practical Diabetes International is published every 2 months. PMH Publications, PO BOX 100, Chichester, West Sussex, PO18 8HD, mail it free on request to health-care professionals
2. Diabetes Digest can be obtained from SB Communications Group, 15 Mandeville Courtyard, 142 Battersea Park Road, London SW11 4NB; telephone 020-7627 1510; e-mail: info@sbcommunicationsgroup.com

Important research and reviews about diabetes may be published in eminent peer-reviewed journals with wide circulation, such as the *British Medical Journal*, the *Lancet*, or *The New England Journal of Medicine*, or those with specialist interest, such as *Diabetes Care*, *Diabetic Medicine*, or *Diabetologica*. These are either available on subscription or are held in most hospital postgraduate libraries.

Electronic resources
Traditional textbooks fail frequently to incorporate newly published research. Electronic evidence databases are regarded as being better able to overcome these drawbacks. No single database will address all needs. A comprehensive search needs to choose an effective strategy that will look at several appropriate databases.

Most local postgraduate medical libraries provide training sessions, well worth investigating. Another invaluable benefit of contacting the library is to obtain a personal ATHENS (Access To Higher Education via NISS authentication System) username and password. This allows the user free access to otherwise remote or pay-to-view electronic resources.

Every effort has been made to ensure that the web addresses cited below are accurate at the time of printing. If these change, browsers may be redirected to the new webpage, or can use a search engine such as Google.

A good starting point is the National electronic Library of Health (NeLH), which is well organised and has excellent links. It is available free both to NHS staff via the NHSNet and to the general public; online: www.nelh.nhs.uk/. The NLH has its diabetes specialist library, online: http://libraries.nelh.nhs.uk/diabetes/.

The following web sites are useful:

- Many, but not all, medical articles are indexed in the massive Medline database, compiled by the National Library of Medicine in the United States. There is no filtering on the original Medline, so each article needs to be evaluated critically. Free access to Medline has been available since 1997 via PubMed, online: http://www.ncbi.nih.gov/entrez/query.fcgi.
- **AMED** (Allied and Complimentary Medicine Database) is a unique bibliographic database produced by the Health Care Information Service of the British Library. It covers a selection of journals in three separate subject areas, several professions allied to medicine, complementary medicine and palliative care. NHS professionals in England and Wales have free access to AMED via the NHSNet. Further details are available, online: http://www.bl.uk/collections/health/amed.html.
- **Clinical Evidence** is an important and useful part of the NeLH. It gathers together the best available evidence on the effects of common clinical interventions. It is available either: electronically on www.clinicalevidence.com (updated monthly) or in a concise paper version published by the BMJ Publishing Group (updated in June and December) and sent free to doctors. This website also has a section aimed at patients: www.besttreatments.com.
- The **Cochrane Library** is a collection of databases, updated quarterly, which include systematic reviews and registers of controlled trials. Many researchers now favour Cochrane when starting a literature search. It can be accessed on the Web: http://www.cochrane.org/index2.htm. The Cochrane Database of Systematic Reviews is an important information source for the effectiveness of treatments. It is available free to NHS staff via the knowledge section of the NeLH and the abstracts are free to all via: http://www.update-software.com/publications/cochrane/.
- Several free related databases are available online: http://www.york.ac.uk/inst/crd/crddatabases.htm
  - **DARE** (the database of abstracts of reviews of effectiveness)
  - **NHS EED** (the NHS economic evaluation database)
  - **HTA** (health technology assessment)

- **TRIP** is a free database that searches over 55 sites of high-quality medical information, online: http://www.tripdatabase.com/. Free access can be obtained by logging in via ATHENS.

Organisations
Many organisations have their own web sites with useful information:

- The *American Diabetes Association* (ADA) publishes comprehensive and referenced clinical practice recommendations that are up-dated annually, available: http://www.diabetes.org.
- The membership of *Diabetes UK* (formerly the British Diabetic Association) includes not only health-care professionals, but also patients and other interested lay people. The address is 10 Parkway, London NW1 7AA, telephone (020) 7424 1000 (GPs and practice nurses can join the Primary Care section). It does post guidance on its website. Online. Available: http://www.diabetes.org.uk.
- The *Primary Care Diabetes Society* (PCDS) was formed in 2005. Its membership is free and includes the whole range of professionals working in primary care with an interest in diabetes. PCDS holds annual conferences and is contactable via its website: http://www.pcdsociety.org/index.htm.
- The *Department of Health* (DoH), for finding official documents: http://www.dh.gov.uk/Home/fs/en.
- *National Institute for Health and Clinical Excellence* (NICE) has guidelines on various aspects of diabetes in support of the Diabetes NSF and on hypertension in 2004, and guidance, particularly on new treatments. Online. Available: http://www.nice.org.uk.
- The *Scottish Intercollegiate Guidelines Network* (SIGN) published in November 2001 its own guidelines for the management of diabetes (guideline number 55). Their evidence base is very well set out and it carries an extensive list of references. They can be downloaded from the SIGN website: http://www.sign.ac.uk/.
- The Science and Education Department of the *British Medical Association* (BMA) produced in 2004 a useful guide for health-care professionals managing patients with diabetes. It is downloadable from the BMA website, online: http://www.bma.org.uk/ap.nsf/Content/Diabetes?OpenDocument&Highlight=2,diabetes.
- The University of Warwick's "*Warwick Diabetes Care*" was launched in 2000. It provides educational courses, support of diabetes research, and practical resources and links. It can be contacted via telephone (024)7657 2958 or e-mail: diabetes@warwick.ac.uk. Its website is http://www2.warwick.ac.uk/fac/med/healthcom/diabetes/.
- The Department of Health's *Medicines and Healthcare products Regulatory Agency* (MHRA) provides information about medical

equipment. Similarly to the yellow card reporting system for adverse drug reactions, the MHRA requests practitioners to report adverse incidents involving medical devices. Obtaining further information or reporting an adverse incident can be done via the MHRA website: www. mhra.gov.uk.

- The *National Diabetes Support Team* (part of the NHS Clinical Governance Support Team) has set up a web forum "to support information exchange and enquiry throughout the diabetes community". It enables people to share their knowledge and experiences of what has either worked or not, online: http://www. diabetes.nhs.uk/forum/.

LIST OF ABBREVIATIONS AND ACRONYMS

4S, Scandinavian Simvastatin Survival Study

AAMI, Association for the Advancement of Medical Instrumentation Standard

ABCD, Appropriate Blood Pressure Control in Diabetes/Association of British Clinical Diabetologists

ABPR, ankle-brachial pressure ratio

ACAT, acyl coenzyme A cholesterol acyltransferase

ACE, angiotensin converting enzyme

ACR, albumin–creatinine ratio

ADA, American Diabetes Association

ADL, Basic Activities of Daily Living

ADDITION, Anglo-Danish-Dutch Study of Intensive Treatment In PeOple with Screen Detected Diabetes IN Primary Care

ADOPT, A Diabetes Outcome Progression Trial

AER, albumin excretion rate

AF, atrial fibrillation

AGEs, advanced glycosylation end products

AIC, Adverse Incident Centre

ALLHAT, **A**ntihypertensive and **L**ipid **L**owering to prevent **H**eart **A**ttack **T**rial

AMED, Allied and Complimentary Medicine Database

ARB, angiotensin II receptor antagonists

ARR, absolute risk reduction

ASCOT, Anglo-Scandinavian Cardiac Outcomes Trial

ASTEROID, **A S**tudy to **E**valuate the Effect of **R**osuvastatin on **I**ntravascular Ultrasound-**D**erived Coronary Atheroma Burden

ATHENS, **A**ccess to **H**igher **E**ducation via **N**ISS Authentication **S**ystem

BHF, British Heart Foundation

BHS, British Hypertension Society

BMA, British Medical Association

BME, black and minority ethnic

BMI, body mass index

BMJ, British Medical Journal

BNF, British National Formulary

CALM, candesartan and lisinopril microalbuminuria

CAN, cardiac autonomic neuropathy

CAPP, Captopril Prevention Project

CARDIA, coronary artery risk development in young adults

CARDS, Collaborative Atorvastatin Diabetes Study

CARE, cholesterol and recurrent events trial

CBT, cognitive behaviour therapy

CCB, calcium channel blocker

CETP, cholesteryl ester transfer protein

CHARM, Candesartan in Heart Failure Assessment of Reduction in Morbidity and mortality
CHD, coronary heart disease
CI, confidence interval
CK, creatine kinase
CNS, central nervous system
CRD, Centre for Reviews and Dissemination
CSMO, clinically significant macular oedema
CVA, cerebrovascular accident
CVD, cardiovascular disease
CPK, creatine phosphokinase
DAFNE, dose adjustment for normal eating
DARE, the database of abstracts of reviews of effectiveness
DASH, Dietary Approaches to Stop Hypertension
DCCB, dihydropyridine calcium channel blocker
DCCT, Diabetes Control and Complications Trial
DECODE, Diabetes Epidemiology: Collaborative Analysis of Diagnostic Criteria in Europe
DESMOND, Diabetes Education for Self-Management: Ongoing and Newly Diagnosed
DoH, Department of Health
DPN, distal symmetric polyneuropathy
DPP, Diabetes Prevention Program
DPP-IV, dipeptidyl peptidase IV
DREAM, Diabetes Reduction Assessment with Ramipril and Rosiglitazone Medication
DSME, diabetes self-management education
DSN, diabetes specialist nurse
DVLA, Driver and Vehicle Licensing Agency
EBM, evidence-based medicine
ECG, electrocardiogram
eGFR, estimated glomerular filtration rate
EHIC, European Health Insurance Card
EMEA, European Agency for the Evaluation of Medicinal Products
EMP, enzyme modification of porcine insulin
EUROPA, EURopean trial On reduction of cardiac events with Perindopril in stable coronary Artery disease
FACET, Fosinopril versus Amlodipine Cardiovascular Events Randomised Trial
FDA, Food and Drug Administration
FIELD, Fenofibrate Intervention and Event Lowering in Diabetes study
g, grams
GDM, gestational diabetes mellitus
GI, glycaemic index OR gastro-intestinal

GLP-1, glucagon-like peptide-1
GMP, guanosine monophosphate
GMS, General Medical Services
GP, general practitioner
GPAQ, General Practice Assessment Questionnaire
GPRD, General Practice Research Database
GPwSI, general practitioner with a special interest
GTT, glucose tolerance test
HAZ, Health Action Zone
HbA1c, Haemoglobin A1c (glycosylated haemoglobin)
HDFP, Hypertension Detection and Follow-up Program
HDL, high-density lipoprotein
HDL-C, high-density lipoprotein cholesterol
HIV, human immunodeficiency virus
HONK, Hyperosmolar nonketotic hyperglycaemic coma
HOPE, Heart Outcomes Prevention Evaluation Study
HOT, Hypertension Optimal Treatment Trial
HTA, health technology assessment
IDDM, insulin-dependent diabetes mellitus
IDF, International Diabetes Federation
IFG, impaired fasting glucose
IGT, impaired glucose tolerance
INVEST, International Verapamil-Trandolapril Study
INR, international normalised ratio
ISA, intrinsic sympathomimetic activity
IT, information technology
JBS, Joint British Societies
LDL, low-density lipoprotein
LDL-C, low-density lipoprotein cholesterol
LFT, liver function test
LIFE, Losartan Intervention for Endpoint reduction in hypertension study
LIPID, Long-Term Intervention with Pravastatin in Ischaemic Disease Study
LV, left ventricle or left ventricular
LVH, left ventricular hypertrophy
MCV, mean corpuscular volume
MHRA, Medicines and Healthcare products Regulatory Agency
MI, myocardial infarction
MIMS, Monthly Index of Medical Specialties
MMSE, Mini Mental State Examination
MNT, medical nutritional therapy
MODY, maturity-onset diabetes of the young
MRC, Medical Research Council
MRFIT, Multiple Risk Factor Intervention Trial
NCEP, National Cholesterol Education Program

NDA, National Diabetes Audit
NeLH, National electronic Library of Health
NHS, National Health Service
NHS EED, the NHS economic evaluation database
NICE, National Institute for Health and Clinical Excellence
NIDDM, non-insulin-dependent diabetes mellitus
NIH, American National Institute of Health
NNT, number needed to treat
NORDIL, NORdic DILtiazem Study
NPfIT, The National Programme for Information Technology
NPH, neutral protamine Hagedorn
NRT, nicotine replacement therapy
NSC, National Screening Committee
NSF, National Service Framework
NTD, neural tube defect
OGTT, oral glucose tolerance test
PBC, practice-based commissioning
PCDS, Primary Care Diabetes Society
PCT, primary care trust
PDE5, phosphodiesterase type-5 inhibitors
PILs, patient information leaflets
PMS, Personal Medical Services
PPAR-γ, peroxisome proliferator-activated receptor-gamma
PPRG, postprandial glucose regulator
prb, proinsulin synthesised by bacteria
PROactive, PROspective PioglitAzone Clinical Trial In MacroVascular Events
PROCAM, PROspective CArdiovascular Munster Study
PROSPER, PROspective Study of Pravastatin in the Elderly at Risk
PVD, peripheral vascular disease
pyr, precursor synthesised by yeast
QALY, Quality Adjusted Life Year
QMAS, Quality Management and Analysis System
QOF, Quality Outcomes Framework
QUIDS, Quality Indicators for Diabetes Services
RAPRIO, reassurance, advice, prescription, referral, investigations, observation
RCGP, Royal College of General Practitioners
RCT, randomised controlled trial
RECORD, Rosiglitazone Evaluated for Cardiac Outcomes and Regulation of Glycaemia in Diabetes study
RIO, Rimonabant in Obesity
RRR, relative risk reduction
SHEP, Systolic Hypertension in the Elderly Program
SIGN, Scottish Intercollegiate Guidelines Network

SLS, selected list scheme
SPARCL, Stroke Prevention by Aggressive Reduction in Cholesterol Levels
SSRI, selective serotonin reuptake inhibitor
STAR, Screening Those at Risk
STOP-2, Swedish Trial in Old Patients with Hypertension
STOP-NIDDM, Study to Prevent NIDDM
SYST-EUR, Systolic Hypertension in Europe Trial
SYST-CHINA, Systolic Hypertension in China
T2ARDIS, Type 2 Diabetes: Accounting for a Major Resource Demand in
   Society in the UK
TC, total cholesterol
TG, triglyceride
TRIP, Turning Research into Practice
TRIPOD, TRoglitazone In Prevention Of Diabetes
TZD, thiazolidinediones
UKADS, United Kingdom Asian Diabetes Study
UKPDS, United Kingdom Prospective Diabetes Study
VALUE, Valsartan Antihypertensive Long-term Use Evaluation
VLCD, very low-calorie diet
VLDL, very low-density lipoprotein
WHO, World Health Organization
WHR, waist–hip ratio
WOSCOPS, West of Scotland Coronary Prevention Study
XENDOS, XENical in the prevention of Diabetes in Obese Subjects

INTRODUCTION

REFERENCES

Audit Commission 2000 Testing times: a review of diabetes services in England and Wales. London: The Audit Commission.

Byrne CD, Wild SH 2000 Diabetes care needs evidence-based interventions to reduce risk of vascular disease (Editorial). BMJ 320: 1554–1555.

Gray A, Raikou M, McGuire A et al 2000 Cost effectiveness of an intensive blood glucose control policy in patients with type 2 diabetes: economic analysis alongside randomised control trial (UKPDS 41). BMJ 320: 1373–1378.

Holman H, Lorig K 2000 Patients as partners in managing chronic disease. BMJ 320: 526–527.

UK Prospective Diabetes Study Group 1998a Effect of intensive blood-glucose control with metformin on complications in overweight patients with type 2 diabetes (UKPDS 34). Lancet 1998; 352: 854–865.

UK Prospective Diabetes Study Group 1998b Intensive blood-glucose control with sulphonylureas or insulin compared with conventional treatment and risk of complications in patients with type 2 diabetes (UKPDS 33). Lancet 352: 837–853.

UK Prospective Diabetes Study Group 1998c Tight blood pressure control and risk of macro vascular and micro vascular complications in type 2 diabetes: (UKPDS 38). BMJ 317: 703–712.

CHAPTER 1

REFERENCES

Abuissa H, Jones PG, Marso SP et al 2005 Angiotensin-converting enzyme inhibitors or angiotensin receptor blockers for prevention of type 2 diabetes: a meta-analysis of randomized clinical trials. J Am Coll Cardiol 46(5): 821–826.

Alberti KGMM, Zimmet PZ for the WHO Consultation 1998 Definition, diagnosis and classification of diabetes mellitus and its complications. Part 1: diagnosis and classification of diabetes mellitus. Provisional report of a WHO Consultation. Diabet Med 15: 539–553.

Amos AF, McCarty DJ, Zimmet P 1997 The rising global burden of diabetes and its complications: estimates and projections to the year 2010. Diabet Med 14: S7–S85.

Beers MH, Porter RS, Jones TV et al (eds) 2006 The Merck Manual of Diagnosis and Therapy, 18th edn. Whitehouse Station: Merck Research Laboratories.

British Diabetic Association, King's Fund, Economists Advisory Group and SmithKline Beecham Pharmaceuticals UK 2000 T2ARDIS: Implications for Seamless Care Provision in Type 2 Diabetes in the UK. Data presented at the Diabetes UK Professional Conference.

Buchanan TA, Xiang AH, Peters RK et al 2005 Preservation of pancreatic β-cell function and prevention of type 2 diabetes by pharmacological treatment of insulin resistance in high-risk Hispanic women. Diabetes 51: 2796–2803.

Carlsson PO, Berne C, Jansson L 1998 Angiotensin II and the endocrine pancreas: effects on islet blood flow and insulin secretion in rats. Diabetologia 41: 127–133.

Carr DB, Ulzschneider KM, Hull RL et al 2004 Intra-abdominal fat is a major determinant of the National Cholesterol Education Program Adult Treatment Panel III criteria for the metabolic syndrome. Diabetes 53(8): 2087–2094.

Chiasson J-L, Josse RG, Gomis R et al for The STOP-NIDDM Trial Research Group 2002 Acarbose for prevention of type 2 diabetes: the STOP-NIDDM randomised trial. Lancet 359: 2072–2077.

Croxson SCM, Price DE, Burden ML et al 1994 The mortality of elderly people with diabetes. Diabet Med 11: 250–252.

Dählof B, Devereux RB, Kjeldsen SE et al for the LIFE study group 2002 Cardiovascular morbidity and mortality in the losartan intervention for endpoint reduction in hypertension study (LIFE): a randomised trial against atenolol. Lancet 359: 995–1003.

Davies MJ, Grenfell A, Day JL 1996 Clinical characteristics and follow-up of subjects with non-insulin-dependent diabetes mellitus diagnosed by screening. Practical Diabetes Int 1996; 13: S42.

Davies MJ, Burden AC, Burden ML 1997 Screening for type 2: increasing evidence that it is necessary. Part 1: should it be done? Practical Diabetes Int 14: 162–164.

Davies MJ 2006 Data presented at the Annual Professional Conference. Birmingham, UK: Diabetes UK. 30 March 2006.

DECODE Study Group on behalf of the European Diabetes Epidemiology Study Group 1999 Glucose tolerance and mortality: comparison of WHO and American Diabetes Association diagnostic criteria. Lancet 354: 617–621.

Department of Health 2002 National Service Framework for Diabetes: Delivery strategy. London: HMSO.

Department of Health 2006 Your Health, Your Care, Your Say: a new direction for community services. London: HMSO. Available online: http://www.dh.gov.uk/PublicationsAndStatistics/Publications/PublicationsPolicyAndGuidance/PublicationsPolicyAndGuidanceArticle/fs/en?CONTENT_ID=4127453&chk=NXIecj

Diabetes in the UK 2004 A report from Diabetes UK.

Diabetes Prevention Program Research Group 2002 Reduction in the incidence of type 2 diabetes with lifestyle intervention or metformin. N Engl J Med 346: 393–403.

Diabetes UK Available online: http://www.diabetes.org.uk/Guide-to-diabetes/Treatment-your-health/Managing-your-weight/Am-I-overweight (Accessed 4 February 2007).

Drake AJ, Smith A, Betts PR et al 2002 Type 2 diabetes in obese white children. Arch Dis Child 86: 207–208.

DREAM (diabetes reduction assessment with ramipril and rosiglitazone medication) Trial investigators; Gerstein HC, Yusuf S, Bosch J et al 2006 Effect of rosiglitazone on the frequency of diabetes in patients with impaired glucose tolerance or impaired fasting glucose: a randomised controlled trial. Lancet 368:1096–1105.

Expert Committee on the Diagnosis and Classification of Diabetes Mellitus 2003 Follow-up report on the diagnosis of diabetes mellitus. Diabetes Care 26: 3160–3167.

Franse LV, Bari MD, Shorr RI et al 2001 Type 2 diabetes in older well-functioning people: who is undiagnosed? Data from the Health, Aging and Body Composition Study. Diabetes Care 24: 2065–2070.

Gillies CL, Abrams KR, Lambert PC et al 2007 Pharmacological and lifestyle interventions to prevent or delay type 2 diabetes in people with impaired glucose tolerance: systematic review and meta-analysis. BMJ 334: 299.

Goodyer E 2006 Data presented at the Annual Professional Conference. Birmingham, UK: Diabetes UK.

Harris MI, Klein R, Welborn TA et al 1992 Onset of type 2 occurs at least 4–7 years before clinical diagnosis. Diabetes Care 15: 815–819.

Houston TK, Person SD, Pletcher MJ et al 2006 Active and passive smoking and development of glucose intolerance among young adults in a prospective cohort: CARDIA study. BMJ 332: 1064–1067.

International Diabetes Federation press release, 14 April 2005. Available online: http://www. idf.org/home/index.cfm?unode=32EF2063-B966-468F-928C-A5682A4E3910

Jonsson B. CODE-2 advisory board 2002 Revealing the cost of type II diabetes in Europe. Diabetologia 45: S5—12.

Julius S, Kjeldsen SE, Weber M et al 2004 Outcomes in hypertensive patients at high cardiovascular risk treated with regimens based on valsartan or amlodipine: the VALUE randomised trial. Lancet 363: 2022–2031.

Kingdom A, Ferguson B 2006 Diabetes Key Facts. Yorkshire and Humber Public Health Observatory.

Lawrence JM, Bennett P, Young A et al 2001 Screening for diabetes in general practice: cross-sectional population study. BMJ 323: 548–551.

Lindstom J, Ilanne-Parikka P, Peltonen M et al 2006 Sustained reduction in the incidence of type 2 diabetes by lifestyle intervention: follow up of the Finnish Diabetes Prevention Study. Lancet 368: 1673–1679.

Morris AD, Boyle DI, MacAlpine R et al 1997 The diabetes audit and research in Tayside Scotland (DARTS) study: electronic record linkage to create a diabetes register. BMJ 315: 524–528.

Newnham A, Ryan R, Khunti K et al 2002 Prevalence of diagnosed diabetes mellitus in general practice in England and Wales, 1994 to 1998. In National Statistics, Health Statistics Quarterly, Vol. 14. London: HMSO. Available online: http://www.statistics.gov.uk

National Institute for Clinical Excellence 2000 Guidance on Rosiglitazone for Type 2 Diabetes Mellitus. London: Department of Health. Available online: http://www.nice.org.uk

National Screening Committee 1998 First report of the National Screening Committee. London: Health Departments of the United Kingdom. Available online: http://bmj. bmjjournals.com/cgi/content/full/322/7292/986/DC1

Padwal R, Majundar SR, Johnson J et al 2005 A systematic review of drug therapy to delay or prevent type 2 diabetes. Diabetes Care 28(3): 736–744.

Pan XR, Li GW, Hu YH et al 1997 Effects of diet and exercise in preventing NIDDM in people with impaired glucose tolerance: the Da Qing IGT and Diabetes Study. Diabetes Care 20: 537–544.

Panzram G 1987 Mortality and survival in type 2 (non-insulin dependent) diabetes mellitus. Diabetologia 30: 123–131.

Reaven GM 1988 Insulin resistance in human disease. Diabetes 37: 1595–1607.

Santoro D, Natali A, Palombo C et al 1992 Effects of chronic angiotensin converting enzyme inhibition on glucose tolerance and insulin sensitivity in essential hypertension. Hypertension 20: 181–191.

Sattar N 2006 Data presented at the Annual Professional Conference. Birmingham, UK: Diabetes UK.

Stratton IM, Adler AI, Neil HAW et al 2000 Association of glycaemia with macrovascular and microvascular complications of type 2 diabetes (UKPDS 35): prospective observational study. BMJ 321: 405–412.

Sundström J, Risérus U, Byberg L et al 2006 Clinical value of the metabolic syndrome for long term prediction of total and cardiovascular mortality: prospective, population based cohort study BMJ; 0: bmj.38766.624097.1Fv2.

The Expert Committee on the Diagnosis and Classification of Diabetes Mellitus 1997 Report of the Expert Committee on the Diagnosis and Classification of Diabetes Mellitus. Diabetes Care 1997; 20: 1183–1197.

The Expert Committee on the Diagnosis and Classification of Diabetes Mellitus 2003a Position Statement: screening for diabetes. Diabetes Care 26(Suppl. 1): S21–S24.

The Expert Committee on the Diagnosis and Classification of Diabetes Mellitus 2003b Report of the Expert Committee on the Diagnosis and Classification of Diabetes Mellitus. Diabetes Care 26(Suppl. 1): S5–S20.

Torgerson JS, Hauptman J, Boldrin MN et al 2004 XENical in the prevention of Diabetes of Obese Subjects (XENDOS) study: a randomized study of orlistat as an adjunct to lifestyle changes for the prevention of type 2 diabetes in obese patients. Diabetes Care 27: 155–161 (erratum in Diabetes Care 2004; 27: 856).

Tuomilehto J, Lindstorm J, Eriksson JG et al for the Finnish Diabetes Prevention Study Group 2001 Prevention of type 2 diabetes mellitus by changes in lifestyle among subjects with impaired glucose tolerance. N Engl J Med 333: 1343–1350.

Turner RC, Millns H, Neil HAW et al 1998 for the United Kingdom Prospective Diabetes Study Group. Risk factors for coronary artery disease in non-insulin-dependent diabetes mellitus: United Kingdom prospective diabetes study (UKPDS 23). BMJ 316: 823–828.

UK Diabetes Information Audit and Benchmarking Service (UKDIABS) 2000 London: Diabetes UK.

UK Prospective Diabetes Study Group 1998a Intensive blood-glucose control with sulphonylureas or insulin compared with conventional treatment and risk of complications in patients with type 2 diabetes (UKPDS 33). Lancet 352: 837–853.

UK Prospective Diabetes Study Group 1998b Tight blood pressure control and risk of macro vascular and micro vascular complications in type 2 diabetes: (UKPDS 38). BMJ 317: 703–712.

Unwin N, Shaw J, Zimmet P, Alberti KGMM 2002 Impaired glucose tolerance and impaired fasting glycaemia: the current status on definition and intervention. Diabet Med 19: 708–723.

Wanless D 2002 Securing Our Future Health: Taking a Long-Term View. London: HM Treasury. Available online: http://www.hm-treasury.gov.uk/Consultations_and_Legislation/wanless/consult_wanless_final.cfm

Wareham D, Griffin SJ 2001 Should we screen for type 2 diabetes? Evaluation against National Screening Committee criteria. BMJ 322: 986–988.

Whincup PH, Gilg JA, Papacosta O et al 2002 Early evidence of ethnic differences in cardiovascular risk: cross-sectional comparison of British South Asian and white children. BMJ 324: 635–638.

WHO/IDF. 2006 Definition and Diagnosis of Diabetes Mellitus and Intermediate Hyperglycaemia. Report of WHO/IDF Consultation. Geneva, Switzerland: World Health Organisation. Available online: http://www.who.int/diabetes/publications/en/

WHO Study Group on Diabetes Mellitus 1985 Diabetes Mellitus. Technical Report Series No. 727. Geneva, Switzerland: WHO.

Wood D, Wray R, Poulter N et al 2005 JBS 2: Joint British Societies' guidelines on prevention of cardiovascular disease in clinical practice. Heart 91(Suppl. 5):1–52.

Wroe CD 1997 Conference Report from the 57th Annual Meeting and Scientific Sessions of the ADA. Practical Diabetes Int 14: 142.

Yorkshire and Humber Public Health Observatory 2005 PBS Diabetes Population Prevalence Model - Phase 2 - Key Findings. Available online: http://www.york.ac.uk/yhpho/documents/pbsdpm/pbs%20phase%202/PBS%20Key%20Findings%20-%20Phase2.pdf

Yusuf S, Gerstein H, Hoogwerf B et al for the HOPE Study Investigators 2001 Ramipril and the development of diabetes. JAMA 286: 1882–1885.

CHAPTER 2

REFERENCES

Ajani UA, Gaziano JM, Lotufo PA et al 2000 Alcohol consumption and risk of coronary heart disease by diabetes status. Circulation 102: 500–505.

Albright A, Franz M, Hornsby G et al 2000 American College of Sports Medicine Position Stand. Exercise and type 2 diabetes. Med Sci Sports Exerc 32: 1345–1360.

American Diabetes Association 1995 Diabetes and exercise: the risk–benefit profile. In: Devlin JT, Ruderman N (eds) The Health Professional's Guide to Diabetes and Exercise. Alexandria, VA: American Diabetes Association, pp. 3–4.

American Diabetes Association 2003 Position Statement. Evidence-based nutrition principles and recommendations for the treatment and prevention of diabetes and related complications. Diabetes Care 26(Suppl. 1): S51–S61.

American Diabetes Association. Clinical Practice Recommendations 2007. Diabetes Care 30: S1–85. Available online: http://www.diabetes.org

An LC, Zhu S-H, Nelson DB et al 2006 Benefits of telephone care over primary care for smoking cessation. Arch Intern Med 166: 536–542.

Beers MH, Berkow R (eds) 1999 The Merck Manual of Diagnosis and Therapy, 17th edn. Whitehouse Station: Merck Research Laboratories.

Buckley J, Holmes J, Mapp G 1999 Exercise on Prescription: Cardiovascular Activity for Health. Oxford, UK: Butterworth-Heinemann.

Christiansen C, Thomsen C, Rasmussen O et al 1996 The acute impact of ethanol on glucose, insulin, triacylglycerol, and free fatty acid responses and insulin sensitivity in type 2 diabetes. Br J Nutr 22: 669–675.

Connor H, Annan F, Bunn E et al for the Nutritional Subcommittee of the Diabetes Care Advisory Committee of Diabetes UK 2003 The implementation of nutritional advice for people with diabetes. Diabetic Medicine 20: 786–807.

DAFNE Study Group 2002 Training in flexible, intensive insulin management to enable dietary freedom in people with type 1 diabetes: dose adjustment for normal eating (DAFNE) randomised controlled trial. BMJ 325: 746–749.

Department of Health 2004 At Least Five a Week: evidence on the impact of physical activity and its relationship to health. A report from the Chief Medical Officer. London: HMSO.

Department of Health 2004 Health Survey for England 2003: Trends. London: Department of Health. Available online: http://www.dh.gov.uk

Department of Health Tobacco Policy. Available online: www.dh.gov.uk/PolicyAndGuidance/HealthAndSocialCareTopics/Tobacco/fs/en

Department of Health, Diabetes UK 2005 Structured Patient Education in Diabetes: Report from the Patient Education Working Group. London: HMSO.

Enright J 1997 Fortnightly review: cognitive behaviour therapy – clinical applications. BMJ 314: 1811–1823.

Expert Panel on Detection, Evaluation, and Treatment of High Blood Cholesterol in Adults 2001 Executive summary of the third report of the National Cholesterol Education Program (NCEP) Expert Panel on Detection, Evaluation, and Treatment of High Blood Cholesterol in Adults (Adult Treatment Panel III). JAMA 285: 2486–2497.

Gask L, Usherwood T 2002 ABC of psychological medicine: the consultation. BMJ 324: 1567–1569.

Ha T, Lean MEJ 1997 Diet and lifestyle modification in the management of non-insulin-dependent diabetes mellitus. In: Pickup JC, Williams G (eds) Textbook of Diabetes, 2nd edn. Oxford, UK: Blackwell Scientific 37.14–37.15.

Hu FB, Stampfer MJ, Solomon C et al 2001 Physical activity and risk for cardiovascular events in diabetic women. Ann Intern Med 134: 96–105.

Hughes JR, Stead LF, Lancaster T 2004 Antidepressants for smoking cessation. The Cochrane Database of Systematic Reviews, Issue 4. Art. No.: CD000031. DOI: 10.1002/14651858. CD000031.pub2.

Kaplan SH, Greenfield S, Ware JE 1989 Assessing the effects of physician-patient interactions on the outcomes of chronic disease. Med Care 27(Suppl. 3): S110–127.

Kinmonth AL, Woodcock A, Griffin S et al 1998 Randomised controlled trial of patient centred care of diabetes in general practice: impact on current wellbeing and future disease risk. The diabetes care from diagnosis research team. BMJ 317: 1202–1208.

Krentz AJ, Bailey CJ 2001 Type 2 Diabetes in Practice. London: Royal Society of Medicine Press Limited.

Lancaster T, Stead L, Silagy C et al for the Cochrane Tobacco Addiction Review Group 2000 Regular review: effectiveness of interventions to help people stop smoking: findings from Cochrane. BMJ 321: 355–358.

Launer J 2002 Narrative-based Primary Care: A Practical Guide. Oxford, UK: Radcliffe Medical Press.

Leicestershire Health 1997: Dietary Recommendations for adults with Diabetes in Leicestershire. Leicestershire: Leicestershire Health Authority.

Macleod CA, Munro J, Brameld K 1994 Health Gain Investment Programme Technical Review Document: Diabetes. Sheffield, UK: Trent Regional Health Authority.

McIntosh A, Hutchinson A, Home PD et al 2002 Clinical Guidelines for Type 2 Diabetes: Blood glucose management. Sheffield, UK: ScHARR, University of Sheffield. Available online: http://www.shef.ac.uk/guidelines/

NHS Health and Social Care Information Centre 2005 Health Survey for England 2004 – updating of trends tables to include 2004 data. Health and Social Care Information Centre. Available online: http://www.ic.nhs.uk/pubs/hlthsvyeng2004upd/2004trendcommentary.pdf/file

NHS Smoking Helpline. Available online: http://www.givingupsmoking.co.uk/

NICE 2003 Guidance on the use of patient education-models for diabetes: technology appraisal 60. London: NHS National Institute for Clinical Excellence. Available online: http://www.nice.org.uk/TA060

NICE 2006a Brief interventions and referral for smoking cessation in primary care and other settings: Public Health Intervention Guidance no.1. London: NHS National Institute for Clinical Excellence. Available online: http://www.nice.org.uk/page.aspx?o=300201

NICE 2006b Four commonly used methods to increase physical activity: brief interventions in primary care, exercise referral schemes, pedometers and community-based exercise programmes for walking and cycling: Public Health Intervention Guidance no.2. London: NHS National Institute for Clinical Excellence. Available online: http://www.nice.org.uk/page.aspx?o=300202

NICE Appraisal Committee 2002 Technology Appraisal Guidance No. 39: Guidance on the use of nicotine replacement therapy (NRT) and bupropion for smoking cessation. London: NHS National Institute for Clinical Excellence. Available online: http://www.nice.org.uk

Pendleton D, Schofield T, Tate P et al 2003 The New Consultation: Developing Doctor–Patient Communication. Oxford, UK: Oxford University Press.

Pierce NS 1999 Diabetes and exercise. Br J Sports Med 33: 161–173.

Prochaska JO, DiClemente CC 1992 Stages of change in the modification of problem behaviors. Prog Behav Modif 28: 183–218.

Richardson P 1998 Psychological treatments. In: Davies T, Craig TKJ (eds) ABC of Mental Health. London: BMJ Books.

Ruderman N, Devlin JT, Schneider SH (eds) 2002 Handbook of Exercise in Diabetes, 2nd edn. Alexandria, VA: American Diabetes Association.

Sacco RL, Elkind M, Boden-Albala B et al 1999 The protective effect of moderate alcohol consumption on ischaemic stroke. JAMA 282: 53–60.

Sacks FM, Svetky LP, Vollmer WM et al 2001 Effects on blood pressure of reduced dietary sodium and the Dietary Approaches to Stop Hypertension (DASH) diet. DASH-Sodium Collaborative Research Group. N Engl J Med 344: 3–10.

Scottish Intercollegiate Guidelines Network 2001 Management of Diabetes: A National Clinical Guideline (Number 55). Edinburgh: SIGN Executive, Royal College of Physicians. Available online: www.sign.ac.uk

Silagy C, Lancaster T, Stead L, Mant D, Fowler G 2004 Nicotine replacement therapy for smoking cessation. The Cochrane Database of Systematic Reviews, Issue 3. Art. No.: CD000146. DOI: 10.1002/14651858.CD000146.pub2.

Stewart MA 1995 Effective physician-patient communication and health outcomes: a review. CMAJ 152: 1423–1433.

Thomas DE, Elliott EJ, Naughton GA 2006 Exercise for type 2 diabetes mellitus. Cochrane Database of Systematic Reviews, Issue 3. Art. No.: CD002968. DOI: 10.1002/14651858. CD002968.pub2.

Toeller M 1993 Diet and diabetes. Diabetes Metab Rev 9(2): 93–108.

Tuomilehto J, Lindstorm J, Eriksson JG et al for the Finnish Diabetes Prevention Study Group 2001 Prevention of type 2 diabetes mellitus by changes in lifestyle among subjects with impaired glucose tolerance. N Engl J Med 333: 1343–1350.

Turner RC, Millns H, Neil HAW et al for the United Kingdom Prospective Diabetes Study Group 1998 Risk factors for coronary artery disease in non-insulin-dependent diabetes mellitus: United Kingdom prospective diabetes study (UKPDS:23). BMJ 316: 823–828.

The University of York-NHS Centre for Reviews and Dissemination 1998 Smoking cessation: What the health service can do. Effectiveness Matters 3(1).

U.S. Department of Health and Human Services 1996 Physical activity and health: A Report of the Surgeon General. Atlanta, GA: U.S. Department of Health and Human Services, Centers for Disease Control and Prevention, National Center for Chronic Disease Prevention and Health Promotion. Available online: http://www.cdc.gov/nccdphp/sgr/pdf/ sgrfull.pdf

Valmadrid CT, Klein R, Moses SE et al 1999 Alcohol intake and the risk of coronary heart disease mortality in persons with older onset diabetes mellitus. JAMA 282: 239–246.

Wei M, Gibbons LW, Kampert JB et al 2000 Low cardiorespiratory fitness and physical inactivity as predictors of mortality in men with type 2 diabetes. Ann Intern Med 132: 605–611.

West R 2005 Smoking: prevalence, mortality and cessation in Great Britain www.rjwest.co.uk/ smokingcessationgb.pdf Updated October 2005; accessed 4 April 2006.

West R 2006 Theory of addiction. Oxford, UK: Blackwells.

West R, Sohal T 2006 "Catastrophic" pathways to smoking cessation: findings from national survey. BMJ 332: 458–460.

Wingard DL, Barrett-Connor E, Wedick E 2002 What is the evidence that changing tobacco use reduces the incidence of diabetic complications? In: Williams R, Herman W, Kinmouth A-L et al (eds) The Evidence Base for Diabetes Care. Chichester, UK: John Wiley & Sons, Ltd.

Zhu SH, Stretch V, Balabanis M et al 1996 Telephone counseling for smoking cessation: effects of single-session and multiple-session interventions. J Consult Clin Psychol 64: 202–211.

CHAPTER 3

REFERENCES

American Diabetes Association 2007 Clinical practice recommendations 2007. Diabetes Care 30: S1–85. Available online: http://www.diabetes.org

Avery L, Moore S 1999 Changing from tablets to insulin (Fact Sheet 13). Diabetes Update.

Bailey CJ, Day C, Krentz A 2003 Nice timing for glitazones. Br J Diab Vasc Dis 3: 308–309.

Capelleri JC, Cafalu JC, Kourides IA et al 2002 Treatment satisfaction in type 2 diabetes: a comparison between an inhaled insulin regimen and a subcutaneous insulin regimen. Clin Ther 24: 552–564.

Chiquette E, Ramirez G, DeFronzo R 2004 A meta-analysis comparing the effect of thiazolidinediones on cardiovascular risk factors. Arch Intern Med 164(19): 2097–2104.

Curley E. Personal communication.

Day C 1996 Thiazolidinediones: a new class of antidiabetic drugs. Diabet Med 16: 179–192.

Dormandy JA, Charbonnel B, Eckland DJA et al 2005 Secondary prevention of macrovascular events in patients with type 2 diabetes in the PROactive Study (PROspective pioglitazone Clinical Trial in macroVascular Events): a randomised controlled trial. Lancet 366: 1279–1289.

Drug and Therapeutics Bulletin 2007; 45: 65–70; doi:10.1136/dtb.2007.45965 Self monitoring of blood glucose in diabetes.

Eurich DT, Majumdar SR, McAlister FA et al 2005 Improved clinical outcomes associated with metformin in patients with diabetes and heart failure. Diabetes Care 28: 2345–2351.

Freemantle N 2005 How well does the evidence on pioglitazone back up researchers' claims for a reduction in macrovascular events? BMJ 331: 836–838.

Higgs ER, Kretz AJ on behalf of the Association of British Clinical Diabetologists 2004 ABCD position statement on glitazones. Pract Diab Internat 27: 293–295.

Home PD, Pocock SJ, Beck-Nielsen H, et al. Rosiglitazone Evaluated for Cardiovascular Outcomes - An Interim Analysis. N Engl J Med. Published online 5 June 2007 (10.1056/NEJMoa073394).

Jones GC, Macklin JP, Alexander WD 2003 Contraindications to the use of metformin (Editorial). BMJ 326: 4–5.

Kahn S, Haffner S, Heise M et al 2006 Glycaemic durability of rosiglitazone, metformin or glyburide monotherapy. N Engl J Med 335: 2427–2443.

Krentz AJ, Bailey CJ 2001 Type 2 Diabetes in Practice. London: Royal Society of Medicine Press Limited.

Krentz AJ, Bailey CJ, Melander A 2000 Thiazolidinediones for type 2 diabetes (Editorial). BMJ 321: 252–253.

Lawton J, Peel E, Douglas M, Parry O 2004 "Urine testing is a waste of time": newly diagnosed type 2 diabetes patients' perceptions of self-monitoring. Diab Med 21: 1045–1048.

MHRA. MHRA statement on cardiac safety of rosiglitazone (brand name Avandia). 23rd May 2007. Online. www.mhra.gov.uk (accessed 3 September 2007)

NICE Appraisal Committee 2002 Technology Guidance Appraisal No. 53: guidance on the use of long-acting insulin analogues for the treatment of diabetes – insulin glargine. London: National Institute for Clinical Excellence. Available online: http://www.nice.org.uk

NICE Appraisal Committee 2003 Technology Guidance Appraisal No. 63: guidance on the use of glitazones for the treatment of type 2 diabetes. London: NHS National Institute for Clinical Excellence. Available online: http://www.nice.org.uk

NICE Guideline Development Group and Recommendations Panel 2002 Inherited Clinical Guideline G. Management of type 2 diabetes: management of blood glucose. London: NHS National Institute for Clinical Excellence. Available online: http://www.nice.org.uk

NICE 2006 National Collaborating Centre for Primary Care and the Centre for Public Health Excellence at NICE. NICE Technology Appraisal Guidance No. 13: inhaled insulin for the treatment of diabetes (types 1 and 2). London: National Institute for Health and Clinical Excellence. Available online: http://www.nice.org.uk/guidance/TA113

National Institute for Health and Clinical Excellence 2006 Inhaled insulin for the treatment of diabetes (types 1 and 2): appraisal consultation documents. Available online: www.nice.org.uk/page.aspx?o=305474 (accessed 7 May).

Nissen SE, Wolski K. Effect of rosiglitazone on the risk of myocardial infarction and death from cardiovascular causes. N Engl J Med Online first. May 21, 2007 (DOI: 10.1056/NEJMoa072761).

Psaty BM, Furberg CD. The record of rosiglitazone and the risk of myocardial infarction. N Engl J Med Published online 5 June 2007.

Richter B, et al. Rosiglitazone for type 2 diabetes mellitus. Cochrane Database of Systematic Reviews 2007, issue 3. Art. No.: CD006063. DOI: 10.1002/14651858.CD006063

Rohlfing CL, Wiedmeyer HM, Little RR et al 2002 Defining the relationship between plasma glucose and HbA1c: analysis of glucose profiles and HbA1c in the Diabetes Control and Complications Trial. Diab Care 25: 275–278.

Salpeter S, Greyber F, Pasternak G et al 2002 Risk of nonfatal lactic acidosis with metformin use in type 2 diabetes mellitus. Cochrane Database Syst Rev 2: CD002967.

UK Prospective Diabetes Study (UKPDS) Group 1998 Intensive blood-glucose control with sulphonylureas or insulin compared with conventional treatment and risk of complications in patients with type II diabetes (UKPDS 33). Lancet 352: 837–853.

Wilbourne J 2002 Administration of insulin by injection. Practical Diabetes Int 19: S1–S4.

CHAPTER 4

REFERENCES

Adler AI, Stratton IM, Neil HAW et al 2000 Association of systolic blood pressure with macrovascular and microvascular complications of type 2 diabetes (UKPDS 36): prospective observational study. BMJ 321: 412–419.

ALLHAT Collaborative Research Group 2000 Major cardiovascular events in hypertensive patients randomized to doxazosin vs chlorthalidone: the Antihypertensive and Lipid-Lowering treatment to prevent Heart Attack Trial (ALLHAT). JAMA 283: 1967–1975.

ALLHAT Collaborative Research Group 2002 Major outcomes in high-risk hypertensive patients randomized to angiotensin-converting enzyme inhibitor or calcium channel blocker vs. diuretic: the Antihypertensive and Lipid-Lowering treatment to prevent Heart Attacks Trial. JAMA 288: 2981–2997.

American Diabetes Association 2004 Position Statement: Aspirin Therapy in Diabetes. Diab Care 27 (Suppl. 1): S72–S73.

American Diabetes Association 2007 Clinical practice recommendations. Diab Care 30: S1–85.

Baigent C, Keech A, Kearney PM et al 2005 Efficacy and safety of cholesterol-lowering treatment: prospective meta-analysis of data from 90 056 participants in 14 randomised trials of statins. Lancet 366: 1267–1278.

Barrett-Connor EL, Cohn BA, Wingard D et al 1991 Why is diabetes mellitus a stronger risk factor for fatal ischemic heart disease in women than in men? The Rancho Bernardo Study. JAMA 265: 627–633.

Betteridge DJ 1997 Lipid disorders in diabetes mellitus. In: Pickup JC, Williams G (eds) Textbook of Diabetes, 2nd edn. Oxford, UK: Blackwell Scientific, Ch 55.

Blood Pressure Lowering Treatment Trialists' Collaboration 2003 Effects of different blood-pressure-lowering regimens on major cardiovascular events: results of prospectively designed overviews of randomised trials. Lancet 362: 1527–1545.

British Hypertension Society website. Available online: http://www.bhsoc.org/how_to_measure_blood_pressure.htm Accessed 30 April 2006.

Brunner E 2006 Oily fish and omega 3 fat supplements. BMJ doi:10.1136/bmj.38798.680185.47 (published 24 March 2006).

Campbell L, Rössner S 2001 Management of obesity in patients with type 2 diabetes. Diab Med 18: 345–354.

Carlberg B, Samuelsson O, Lindholm LH 2004 Atenolol in hypertension: is it a wise choice? Lancet 364: 1684–1689.

Clinical Evidence. Available. Online: www.clinicalevidence.com

Colhoun HM, Betteridge DJ, Durrington PN et al 2004 Primary prevention of cardiovascular disease with atorvastatin in type 2 diabetes in the Collaborative Atorvastatin Diabetes Study (CARDS): a randomised placebo-controlled trial. Lancet 364: 685–696.

Collins R, Armitage J, Parish S et al for the Heart Protection Study Collaborative Group 2002 MRC/BHF Heart Protection Study of cholesterol lowering with simvastatin in 20 536 high-risk individuals: a randomised placebo-controlled trial. Lancet 360: 9326: 7–22 (6 July).

Connor H, Annan F, Bunn E et al for the Nutritional Subcommittee of the Diabetes Care Advisory Committee of Diabetes UK 2003 The implementation of nutritional advice for people with diabetes. Diab Med 20: 786–807.

Connor J, Rafter N, Rodgers A 2004 Do fixed-dose combination pills or unit-of-use packaging improve adherence: a systematic review. Bulletin of the World Health Organization 82(12): 935–939.

Costa J, Borges M, David C et al 2006 Efficacy of lipid lowering drug treatment for diabetic and non-diabetic patients: meta-analysis of randomised controlled trials. BMJ 332: 1115–1118.

Dählof B, Devereux RB, Kjeldsen SE et al for the LIFE study group 2002 Cardiovascular morbidity and mortality in the Losartan Intervention For Endpoint reduction in hypertension study (LIFE): a randomised trial against atenolol. Lancet 359: 995–1003.

Dahlöf B, Sever PS, Poulter NR et al for the ASCOT Investigators 2005 Prevention of cardiovascular events with an antihypertensive regimen of amlodipine adding perindopril as required versus atenolol adding bendroflumethiazide as required, in the Anglo-Scandinavian Cardiac Outcomes Trial-Blood Pressure Lowering Arm (ASCOT-BPLA): a multicentre randomised controlled trial. Published online 4 September 2005. www.thelancet.com DOI:10.1016/S0140-6736(05)67185-1

Dawson KG, McKenzie JK, Ross SA et al 1993 Hypertension and diabetes. Can Med Assoc J 149: 821–826.

Department of Health website: Obesity care pathway. Available online: http://www.dh.gov.uk/PublicationsAndStatistics/Publications/PublicationsPolicyAndGuidance/PublicationsPolicyAndGuidanceArticle/fs/en?CONTENT_ID=4134408&chk=Sq/wNd Accessed 23 May 2006.

Derosa G, Cicero AE, Bertone G et al 2004 Comparison of fluvastatin + fenofibrate combination therapy and fluvastatin monotherapy in the treatment of combined hyperlipidemia, type 2 diabetes mellitus, and coronary heart disease: a 12-month randomized, double-blind, controlled trial. Clin Ther 26: 1599–1607.

Despres J-P, Lemieur I, Prud'homme D 2001 Treatment of obesity: need to focus on high risk abdominally obese patients. BMJ 322: 716–720.

Diabetes UK Care recommendation 2001 Aspirin treatment in Diabetes. Issued April 2001, updated 2004. Available online: http://www.diabetes.org.uk/infocentre/carerec/aspirin.htm

Drugs and Therapeutics Bulletin 2006 Statins for primary prevention in type 2 diabetes. 44(8): 57–59.

Eliasson E 2006 Ethnicity and adverse drug reactions. BMJ 332: 1163–1164.

Estacio RO, Jeffers BW, Hiatt WR et al 1998 The effect of nisoldipine as compared with enalapril on cardiovascular events in patients with non-insulin-dependent diabetes and hypertension. N Engl J Med 338: 645–652.

Goldberg RB, Mellies MJ, Sacks FM et al 1998 Cardiovascular events and their reduction with pravastatin in diabetic and glucose-intolerant myocardial infarction survivors with average cholesterol levels: subgroup analyses in the cholesterol and recurrent events (CARE) trial. The Care Investigators. Circulation 98: 2513–2519.

Grundy SM, Vega GL, McGovern ME et al 2002 Efficacy, safety, and tolerability of once-daily niacin for the treatment of dyslipidemia associated with type 2 diabetes: results of the assessment of diabetes control and evaluation of the efficacy of niaspan trial (AVENT). Arch Intern Med 162: 1568–1576.

Heart Outcomes Prevention Evaluation Study Investigators 2000 Effects of ramipril on cardiovascular and microvascular outcomes in patients with diabetes mellitus: results of the HOPE study and the MICRO-HOPE study. Lancet 355: 253–259.

Heart Protection Study Collaborative Group 2003 MRC/BHF Heart Protection Study of cholesterol-lowering with simvastatin in 5963 people with diabetes: a randomised placebo-controlled trial. Lancet 361: 2005–2016.

Heinonen OP, Huttunen JK, Manninen V et al 1994 The Helsinki Heart Study: coronary heart disease incidence during an extended follow-up. J Intern Med 235: 41–49.

Hood S, Cannon J, Foo R et al 2002 High prevalence of aldosterone-sensitive hypertension in unselected patients. Q J Medicine 95: 621.

Hooper L, Thompson RL, Harrison RA et al 2006 Risks and benefits of omega 3 fats for mortality, cardiovascular disease, and cancer: systematic review. BMJ doi:10.1136/bmj.38755.366331.2F (published 24 March 2006).

Hutchinson A, McIntosh A, Griffiths CJ et al 2002 Clinical Guidelines and Evidence Review for Type 2 Diabetes. Blood pressure management. Sheffield, UK: ScHARR, University of Sheffield. Available online: http://shef.ac.uk/guidelines

Huxley R, Barzi F, Woodward M 2006 Excess risk of fatal coronary heart disease associated with diabetes in men and women: meta-analysis of 37 prospective cohort studies. BMJ 332: 73–76.

Keech A, Simes RJ, Barter P et al 2005 Effects of long-term fenofibrate therapy on cardiovascular events in 9795 people with type 2 diabetes mellitus (the FIELD study): randomised controlled trial. Lancet 366: 1849–1861.

Koskinen P, Manttair M, Manninen V et al 1992 Coronary heart disease incidence in NIDDM patients in the Helsinki Heart Study. Diabetes Care 15: 820–825.

Law MR, Wald NJ 2002 Risk factor thresholds: their existence under scrutiny. BMJ 324: 1370–1376 (29 June).

Leicestershire Health 1997 Dietary Recommendations for Adults with Diabetes in Leicestershire. Leicester, UK: Leicestershire Health.

Lindholm LH, Ibsen H, Dahlof B et al 2002 Cardiovascular morbidity and mortality in patients with diabetes in the Losartan Intervention For Endpoint reduction in hypertension study (LIFE): a randomised trial against atenolol. Lancet 359: 1004–1010.

Long-Term Intervention with Pravastatin in Ischaemic Disease (LIPID) Study Group 1998 Prevention of cardiovascular events and death with pravastatin in patients with coronary heart disease and a broad range of initial cholesterol levels. N Engl J Med 339: 1349–1357.

Luft FC 2001 Mechanisms and cardiovascular damage in hypertension. Hypertension 37: 594–598.

Maier C, Mustapic D, Schuster E et al 2006 Effect of a pocket-sized tablet dispensing device on patients' glycaemic control in type 2 diabetic patients. Diab Med 23(1): 40–45.

Mancia G, Brown M, Castaigne A et al and INSIGHT 2003 Outcomes with nifedipine GITS or Co-amilozide in hypertensive diabetics and nondiabetics in Intervention as a Goal in Hypertension (INSIGHT). Hypertension 41: 431–436.

Marshall SM, Flyvbjerg A 2006 Prevention and early detection of vascular complications of diabetes. BMJ 333: 475–480.

McDowell S, Coleman JJ, Ferner RE 2006 Systematic review and meta-analysis of ethnic differences in risks of adverse reactions to drugs used in cardiovascular medicine. BMJ 332: 1177–1181.

McIntosh A, Hutchinson A, Feder G et al. Clinical Guidelines and Evidence Review for Type 2 Diabetes. Lipids management. Sheffield, UK: ScHARR, University of Sheffield, 2002. Available online: http://shef.ac.uk/guidelines

Medicines and Healthcare products Regulation Agency 2006 Measuring Blood Pressure – Top Ten Tips. Available online: http://www.mhra.gov.uk

Mogensen CE, Neldam S, Tikkansen I et al 2000 for the CALM study group. Randomised control trial of dual blockade of the rennin-angiotensin system in patients with hypertension, microalbuminuria, and non-insulin dependent diabetes: the candesartan and lisinopril microalbuminuria (CALM) study. BMJ 321: 1440–1444.

New Zealand Guidelines Group (NZGG 2003 The assessment and management of cardiovascular risk. Available online: http://www.nzgg.org.nz/guidelines/0035/CVD_Risk_Full.pdf

NICE 2006 National Collaborating Centre for Primary Care and the Centre for Public Health Excellence at NICE. NICE technology appraisal guidance 113. Inhaled insulin for the treatment of diabetes (types 1 and 2). London: National Institute for Health and Clinical Excellence. Available online: http://www.nice.org.uk/guidance/TA113.

NICE Appraisal Committee 2002 Technology Appraisal Guidance No. 46: the clinical effectiveness and cost effectiveness of surgery for people with morbid obesity. London: NHS National Institute for Clinical Excellence. Available online: http://www.nice.org.uk/page.aspx?o=TA046

NICE 2006a Management of hypertension in adults in primary care: NICE clinical guideline 34. London: NHS National Institute for Clinical Excellence. Available online: http://www.nice.org.uk/page.aspx?o=CG034fullguideline

NICE 2006b Statins for the prevention of cardiovascular events: technology Appraisal 94. London: NHS National Institute for Clinical Excellence. Available online: http://www.nice.org.uk/TA094

Nissen SE, Nichols SJ, Sipahi I et al 2006 Effect of Very High-Intensity Statin Therapy on Regression of Coronary Atherosclerosis: the ASTEROID Trial. JAMA 295: (doi:10.1001/jama.295.13.jpc60002). Available online: http://jama.ama-assn.org/

North of England Hypertension Guideline Development Group 2004 Evidence-based Clinical Practice Guideline: Essential hypertension: managing adults in primary care. London: HMSO National Institute of Clinical Excellence.

O'Brien E, Beevers G, Lip GYH 2001 ABC of hypertension. Blood pressure measurement. Part IV. Automated sphygmomanometry: self blood pressure measurement. BMJ 322: 1167–1170.

O'Brien E, Asmar R, Beilin L et al 2003 European Society of Hypertension Working Group on Blood Pressure Monitoring. European Society of Hypertension recommendations for conventional, ambulatory and home blood pressure measurement. J Hypertension 21: 821–848.

Pepine CJ, Handberg EM, Cooper-De-Hoff RM et al 2003 A calcium antagonist vs. a non-calcium antagonist hypertension treatment strategy for patients with coronary artery disease: the International Verapamil-Trandolapril Study (INVEST): a randomized controlled trial. JAMA 290: 2805–2816.

Pfeffer MA, Swedberg K, Granger CB et al 2003 Effects of candesartan on mortality and morbidity in patients with chronic heart failure: the CHARM-Overall programme. Lancet 362: 759–766.

Pi-Sunyer FX, Aronne LJ, Heshmati HM et al for the RIO-North America Study Group 2006 Effect of rimonabant, a cannabinoid-1 receptor blocker, on weight and cardiometabolic risk factors in overweight or obese patients: RIO-North America: a randomized controlled trial. JAMA 295(7): 761–775.

PROGRESS group 2001 Randomised trial of a perindopril-based blood-pressure-lowering regimen among 6,105 individuals with previous stroke or transient ischaemic attack. Lancet 358: 1033–1041.

Ramsay LE, Williams B, Johnston GD et al 1999 British Hypertension Society guidelines for hypertension management 1999: summary. BMJ 319: 630–635.

Reckless JPD 2006 Diabetes and lipid lowering: where are we? BMJ 332: 1103–1104.

Rubins HB, Robins SJ, Collins D et al 1999 Gemfibrozil for the secondary prevention of coronary heart disease in men with low levels of high-density lipoprotein cholesterol: Veterans Affairs High-Density Lipoprotein Cholesterol Intervention Trial Study Group. N Engl J Med 341: 410–418.

Scandinavian Simvastatin Survival Study 1994 Randomised trial of cholesterol lowering in 4444 patients with coronary heart disease: the Scandinavian Simvastatin Survival Study (4S). Lancet 344: 1383–1389.

Scottish Intercollegiate Guidelines Network (SIGN) 1997. Management of Diabetic Cardiovascular Disease, 1–22. Available online: http://www.sign.ac.uk

Sever PS, Dahlof B, Poulter NR et al; ASCOT investigators 2003 Prevention of coronary and stroke events with atorvastin in hypertensive patients who have average or lower-than-average cholesterol concentrations, in the Anglo-Scandinavian Cardiac Outcomes Trial–Lipid Lowering Arm (ASCOT-LLA): a multicenter randomized controlled trial. Lancet 361: 1149–1158.

Shepherd J, Blauw GJ, Murphy MB et al 2002 Pravastatin in elderly individuals at risk of vascular disease (PROSPER): a randomised controlled trial. Lancet 360:1623–1630.

Simmons D 2002 Prevention of complications: a commentary. In: Williams R, Herman W, Kinmouth A-L et al (eds). The Evidence Base for Diabetes Care. Chichester, UK: John Wiley & Sons, Ltd.

Simons L, Tonkon M, Masana L et al 2004 Effects of ezetimibe added to on-going statin therapy on the lipid profile of hypercholesterolemic patients with diabetes mellitus or metabolic syndrome. Curr Med Res Opin 20: 1437–1445.

Sjöström L, Lindroos A-K, Peltonen M et al 2004 Lifestyle, diabetes, and cardiovascular risk factors 10 years after bariatric surgery. N Engl J Med 351: 2683–2693.

Stamler J, Vaccaro O, Neaton JD, Wentworth D 1993 Diabetes, other risk factors, and 12-yr cardiovascular mortality for men screened in the Multiple Risk Factor Intervention Trial. Diab Care 16: 433–444.

Stevens RJ, Kothari V, Adler AI, Stratton IM, Holman RR on behalf of the United Kingdom Prospective Diabetes Study (UKPDS) Group 2001 The UKPDS risk engine: a model for the risk of coronary heart disease in Type II diabetes (UKPDS 56). Clin Sci 101: 671–679.

Stratton IM, Adler AI, Neil HAW et al 2000 Association of glycaemia with macrovascular and microvascular complications of type 2 diabetes (UKPDS 35): prospective observational study. BMJ 321: 405–412.

Tatti P, Pahor M, Byington PB et al 1998 Outcome results of the Fosinopril Versus Amlodipine Cardiovascular Events Randomized Trial (FACET) in patients with hypertension and NIDDM. Diab Care 21: 597–603.

Turner RC, Millns H, Neil HAW et al 1998 Risk factors for coronary artery disease in non-insulin dependent diabetes mellitus. United Kingdom Prospective Diabetes Study (UKPDS 23). BMJ 316: 823–828.

UK Prospective Diabetes Study Group 1998a Efficacy of atenolol and captopril in reducing risk of macro vascular and micro vascular complications in type 2 diabetes: (UKPDS 39). BMJ 317: 713–720.

UK Prospective Diabetes Study Group 1998b Tight blood pressure control and risk of macro vascular and micro vascular complications in type 2 diabetes: (UKPDS 38). BMJ 317: 703–712.

University of York Centre for Reviews and Dissemination 1994 Effective health care: effectiveness of antihypertensive drugs in black people. 8 (4). Available online: http://www.york.ac.uk/inst/crd/ehc84.pdf

Van Gaal LF, Rissanen AM, Scheen AJ et al for the RIO-Europe Study Group 2005 Effects of the cannabinoid-1 receptor blocker rimonabant on weight reduction and cardiovascular risk factors in overweight patients: 1-year experience from the RIO-Europe study. Lancet 365: 1389–1397.

Verhamme K, Mosis G, Dielman J et al 2006 Spironolactone and risk of upper gastrointestinal events: population based case-control study. BMJ 333: 330–333.

Whelton PK, Barzilay J, Cushaman WC et al 2005 Clinical outcomes in antihypertensive treatment of type 2 diabetes, impaired fasting glucose concentration, and normoglycemia: Antihypertensive and Lipid-Lowering treatment to prevent Heart Attack Trial (ALLHAT). Archiv Intern Med 165: 1410–1419.

Williams B, Poulter NR, Brown MJ et al. Guidelines for management of hypertension: report of the fourth working party of the British Hypertension Society, 2004 BHS iv. J Hum Hypertension 2004: 18: 139–185.

Winocour PH 2002 Effective diabetes care: a need for realistic targets. BMJ 324: 1577–1580 (29 June).

Winocour PH, Fisher M 2003 Prediction of cardiovascular risk in people with diabetes. Diab Med 20: 515–527.

Wood D, Wray R, Poulter N et al 2005 JBS 2: Joint British Societies' guidelines on prevention of cardiovascular disease in clinical practice. Heart 91(Suppl. 5):1–52.

WOSCOPS 1998 Influence of pravastatin and plasma lipids on clinical events in the West of Scotland Coronary Prevention Study (WOSCOPS). Circulation 97: 1440–1445.

Wright EC. Non-compliance – or how many aunts has Matilda? Lancet 1993; 342: 909–913.

CHAPTER 5

REFERENCES

AACE Male Sexual Dysfunction Task Force 2003 American Association of Clinical Endocrinologists medical guidelines for clinical practice for the evaluation and treatment of male sexual dysfunction: a couple's problem – 2003 update. Endocr Pract 9: 77–95.

American Diabetes Association 2007 Clinical practice recommendations 2007. Diabetes Care 30: S1–S85. Available online: http://www.diabetes.org

Atiemo HO, Szostak MJ, Sklar GN 2003 Salvage of sildenafil failures referred from primary care physicians. J Urol 170: 2356–2358.

Barnett AH, Bain SC, Bouter P et al 2004 Angiotensin-receptor blockade versus converting-enzyme inhibition in type 2 diabetes and nephropathy. N Engl J Med 351: 1952–1961.

Black HR, Elliott WJ, Grandits G et al 2003 Principal results of the Controlled Onset Verapamil Investigation of Cardiovascular End Points (CONVINCE) trial. JAMA 289: 2073–2082.

Boulton AJM 1997 The diabetic foot. Medicine 25: 39–42.

Brenner BM, Cooper ME, de Zeeuw D et al 2001 Effects of losartan on renal and cardiovascular outcomes in patients with type 2 diabetes and nephropathy. N Engl J Med 345: 861–869.

Clinical Evidence. Available online: http://www.clinicalevidence.com

Davies TME, Millns H, Stratton IM et al 1999 Risk factors for stroke in non-insulin dependent diabetes mellitus: (UKPDS 29). Arch Intern Med 159: 1097–1103.

DoH Renal NSF Team 2005 The National Service Framework for Renal Services. Part 2: chronic kidney disease, acute renal failure and end of life care. London: Department of Health. Available online: http://www.dh.gov.uk/assetRoot/04/10/26/80/04102680.pdf (Accessed April 2006).

Dinneen SF, Gerstein HC 1997 The association of microalbuminuria and mortality in non-insulin-dependent diabetes mellitus. Arch Intern Med 157: 1413–1418.

Ebskov B, Josephsen P 1980 Incidence of reamputation and death after gangrene of the lower extremity. Prosthet Orthot Int 4: 77–80.

Edmonds ME, Blundell MP, Morris ME et al. Improved survival of the diabetic foot: the role of the specialised foot clinic. Quart J Med 60: 763–771.

Eisenberg E, McNicol E, Carr DB 2006 Opioids for neuropathic pain. Cochrane Database of Systematic Reviews, Issue 3. Art. No.: CD006146. DOI: 10.1002/14651858.CD006146.

Evans J, Rooney C, Ashwood F et al 1996 Blindness and partial sight in England and Wales: April 1990-March 1991. Health Trends 28: 5–12.

Feldman HA, Goldstein I, Hatzichristou DG et al 1994 Impotence and its medical and psychosocial correlates: results of the Massachusetts Male Aging Study. J Urol 151: 54–61.

Gaede P, Vedel P, Larsen N et al 2003 Multifactorial intervention and cardiovascular disease in patients with type 2 diabetes. N Engl J Med 348: 383–393.

Hutchinson A, McIntosh A, Peters J et al 2001 Clinical Guidelines for Type 2 Diabetes: Diabetic retinopathy: early management and screening. Sheffield, UK: ScHARR, University of Sheffield. Available online: http://www.shef.ac.uk/guidelines/

Klein R, Klein BE, Moss SE et al 1984 The Wisconsin epidemiologic study of diabetic retinopathy III. Prevalence and risk of diabetic retinopathy when age at diagnosis is 30 or more years. Arch Ophthalmol 102: 527–532.

Krans HMJ, Porta M, Keen H et al (eds) 1995 Diabetes Care and Research in Europe. The St Vincent Declaration Action Programme Implementation Document, 2nd edn. Copenhagen, Denmark: World Health Organization, Regional Office for Europe.

Kumar S, Ashe HA, Parnell LN et al 1994 The prevalence of foot ulceration and its correlates in type 2 diabetic patients. Diabet Med 11: 480–484.

Laing SP, Swerdlow AJ, Carpenter LM et al 2003 Mortality from heart disease in a cohort of 23000 patients with insulin-treated diabetes. Diabetologia 46: 760–765.

Leicestershire Health 1996 The Leicestershire Handbook for Diabetes, Leicester, UK: Leicestershire Health Authority.

Levene LS, McNally PG, Fraser RC, Lowy AGJ 2004 What characteristics are associated with screening positive for microalbuminuria in patients with diabetes in the community? Pract Diab Internat 21: 287–292.

Levey A, Bosch J, Lewis JB, Greene T, Rogers N, Roth D 1999 A more accurate method to estimate glomerular filtration rate from serum creatinine: a new prediction equation. Ann Intern Med 130: 461–470.

Lewis EJ, Hunisicker I G, Clarke WR et al 2001 Renoprotective effect of the angiotensin-receptor antagonist irbesartan in patients with nephropathy due to type 2 diabetes. N Engl J Med 345: 851–860.

Lip GYH, Kamath S, Freestone B 2003 Acute atrial fibrillation. Clin Evid 8. Available online (free to NHS staff via the National Electronic Library of Health): http://www.nelh.nhs.uk/clinical_evidence.asp

Macleod AF 1997 Diabetic neuropathy. Medicine 25: 36–38.

Macleod CA, Munro J, Brameld K 1994 Health Gain Investment Programme Technical Review Document: Diabetes. Sheffield, UK: Trent Regional Health Authority.

MacLeod JM, Lutale J, Marshall SM 1995 Albumin excretion and vascular deaths in NIDDM. Diabetologia 38: 610–616.

Marshall SM, Flyvbjerg A 2006 Prevention and early detection of vascular complications of diabetes. BMJ 333: 475–480.

Mason L, Moore RA, Derry S, Edwards JE, McQuay HJ 2004 Systematic review of topical capsaicin for the treatment of chronic pain. BMJ 328: 991.

McCullough AR, Barada JH, Fawzy A et al 2002 Achieving treatment optimisation with sildenafil citrate (Viagra) in patients with erectile dysfunction. Urology 60(Suppl.): 28.

McIntosh A, Peters J, Young R et al 2003 Prevention and Management of Foot Problems in Type 2 diabetes: Clinical Guidelines and Evidence. Sheffield, UK: University of Sheffield. Available online: http://www.nice.org.uk

McMahon CN, Smith CJ, Shabsigh R 2006 Practice pointer: treating erectile dsyfunction when PDE5 inhibitors fail. BMJ 332: 589–592.

NICE Guideline Development Group and Recommendations Panel 2002a Inherited Clinical Guideline E. Management of type 2 diabetes: retinopathy – screening and early management. London: NHS National Institute for Clinical Excellence. Available online: http://www.nice.org.uk

NICE Guideline Development Group and Recommendations Panel 2002b Inherited Clinical Guideline F. Management of type 2 diabetes: renal disease – prevention and early management. London: NHS National Institute for Clinical Excellence. Available online: http://www.nice.org.uk

O'Meara SO, Nelson EA, Golder S et al on the behalf of the DASIDU Steering Group 2006 Systematic review of methods to diagnose infection in foot ulcers in diabetes. Diabetic Medicine 23: 341–347.

Parving HH, Lehnert H, Brochner-Mortensen J et al 2001 The effect of irbesartan on the development of diabetic nephropathy in patients with type 2 diabetes. N Engl J Med 345: 870–878.

Pepine CJ, Handberg EM, Cooper-De-Hoff RM et al 2003 A calcium antagonist vs. a non-calcium antagonist hypertension treatment strategy for patients with coronary artery disease: the International Verapamil-Trandolapril Study (INVEST): a randomized controlled trial. JAMA 290: 2805–2816.

Ralph D, McNicholas T for the Erectile Dysfunction Alliance 2000 UK management guidelines for erectile dysfunction. BMJ 321: 409–503.

Roderick PJ, Raleigh VS, Hallam L, Mallick NP 1996 The need and demand for renal replacement therapy in ethnic minorities in England. J Epidemiol Community Health 50: 334–339.

Saarto T, Wiffen PJ 2005 Antidepressants for neuropathic pain. The Cochrane Database of Systematic Reviews, Issue 3. Art. No.: CD005454. DOI: 10.1002/14651858.CD005454.

Savage S, Estacio RO, Jeffers B et al 1996 Urinary albumin excretion as a predictor of diabetic retinopathy, neuropathy and cardiovascular disease in NIDDM. Diabetes Care 19: 1243–1248.

Stratton IM, Adler AI, Neil HAW et al 2000 Association of glycaemia with macrovascular and microvascular complications of type 2 diabetes (UKPDS 35): prospective observational study. BMJ 321: 405–412.

Strippoli GF, Craig M, Craig JC 2005 Antihypertensive agents for preventing diabetic kidney disease. Cochrane Database Syst Rev 4: CD004136.

Tesfaye S, Kempler P 2005 Painful diabetic neuropathy. Diabetologia 48: 805–807.

UK National Screening Committee 2004 Essential Elements in Developing a Diabetic Retinopathy Screening Programme workbook, version 3.2, October 2004. Available online: http://www.nscretinopathy.org.uk/pages/nsc.asp?ModT=A&Sec=16

UK Prospective Diabetes Study (UKPDS) Group 1998a Effect of intensive blood-glucose control with metformin on complications in overweight patients with type 2 diabetes (UKPDS 34). Lancet 352: 854–865.

UK Prospective Diabetes Study (UKPDS) Group 1998b Intensive blood-glucose control with sulphonylureas or insulin compared with conventional treatment and risk of complications in patients with type 2 diabetes (UKPDS 33). Lancet 352: 837–853.

UK Prospective Diabetes Study (UKPDS) Group 1998c Tight blood pressure control and risk of macro vascular and micro vascular complications in type 2 diabetes: (UKPDS 38). BMJ 317: 703–712.

Wagner FW 1983 Algorithms of diabetic foot care. In: Levin ME, O'Neil LW (eds). The Diabetic Foot, 2nd edn. St Louis, MO: Mosby-Yearbook, pp. 291–302.

Wong M-C, Chung JWY, Wong TKS. Effects of treatments for symptoms of painful diabetic neuropathy: systematic review. Br Med J 2007; 335: 87–90. Online: http://www.bmj.com/cgi/content/full/335/7610/87

CHAPTER 6

REFERENCES

Ali S, Stone MA, Peters JL et al 2006 The prevalence of comorbid depression in adults with type 2 diabetes: a systematic review and meta-analysis. Diabetic Medicine 23: 1165–1173.

American Diabetes Association. Clinical practice recommendations 2007 Diabetes Care 2007; 30: S1–85. Available online: http://www.diabetes.org

Anderson RJ, Freedland KE, Clouse RE et al 2001 The prevalence of comorbid depression in adults with diabetes: a meta-analysis. Diabetes Care 24(6): 1069–1078.

Audit Commission 2000 Testing times: a review of diabetes services in England and Wales. London: Audit Commission.

British Heart Foundation 2001 Coronary heart disease. Statistics: Diabetes Supplement. London: BHF.

Ceysens G, Rouiller D, Boulvain M 2006 Exercise for diabetic pregnant women. Cochrane Database of Systematic Reviews, Issue 3. Art. No.: CD004225. DOI: 10.1002/14651858. CD004225.pub2.

Department of Health/Diabetes UK 2005 Care recommendation – recommendations for the management of pregnant women with diabetes (including Gestational diabetes). Updated June. Available online: http://www.diabetes.org.uk/hcpreports/carerecs.htm (Accessed February 2006).

Diabetes UK Insurance Services. Available online: http://www.diabetes.org.uk/services/travel.htm (Accessed 1 May 2006).

DVLA http://www.dvla.gov.uk/at_a_glance/ch3_diabetes.htm (Accessed 1 May 2006).

Gilbody S, Sheldon T, Wessely S 2006 Should we screen for depression? BMJ 332: 1027–1030.

Goldney RD, Phillips PJ, Fisher LJ et al 2004 Diabetes, depression, and quality of life: a population study. Diabetes Care 27(5): 1066–1070.

Hughes RC, Rowan JA 2006 Pregnancy in women with type 2 diabetes: who takes metformin and what is the outcome. Diabetic Medicine 23: 318–322.

Knutsson A 2003 Health disorders of shift workers. Occup Med 53: 103–108.

Lustman PJ, Griffith LS, Freedland KE et al 1988 Cognitive behaviour therapy for depression in type 2 diabetes mellitus. A randomized, controlled trial. Ann Intern Med 129: 613–621.

Lustman PJ, Freedland KE, Griffith LS et al 2000 Fluoxetine for depression in diabetes: a randomized double-blind placebo-controlled trial. Diabetes Care 236: 618–623.

O'Hare JP, Raymond NT, Mughal S et al 2004 Evaluation of delivery of enhanced diabetes care to patients of South Asian ethnicity: the United Kingdom Asian Diabetes Study (UKADS). Diabetic Medicine 21(12): 1357–1365.

CHAPTER 7

REFERENCES

American Diabetes Association 2007 Clinical practice recommendations 2007. Diabetes Care 30: S1–S85. Online: http://www.diabetes.org

Baker R, Fraser RC 1995 Development of audit criteria: linking guidelines and assessment of quality. BMJ 31: 370–373.

Brown AF, Mangione CM, Saliba D et al 2003 Guidelines for improving the care of the older person with diabetes mellitus. J Am Geriatr Soc 51: S265–S280.

Choe HM, Mitrovich S, Dubay D et al 2005 Proactive case management of high risk patients with type 2 diabetes mellitus by a clinical pharmacist: a randomized controlled trial. Am J Manag Care 11: 253–260.

Department of Health 1998 A First Class Service. London: Department of Health.

Department of Health 2001 National Service Framework for Diabetes: Standards. London: HMSO.

Department of Health 2002 National Service Framework for Diabetes: Delivery strategy. London: HMSO.

Department of Health 2003 Diabetes Information Strategy. London: Department of Health. Online: http://www.doh.gov.uk/ipu/strategy/nsf/dis.pdf.

Department of Health 2006 Your Health, Your Care, Your Say: a new direction for community services. London: HMSO. Available online: http://www.dh.gov.uk/PublicationsAndStatistics/Publications/PublicationsPolicyAndGuidance/PublicationsPolicyAndGuidanceArticle/fs/en?CONTENT_ID=4127453&chk=NXIecj

DH Renal NSF Team 2005 The National Service Framework for Renal Services, Part 2: Chronic Kidney Disease, Acute Renal Failure and End of Life Care. London: HMSO.

Diabetes UK 2000 Recommendations for the Management of Diabetes in Primary Care, 3rd edn. London: Diabetes UK.

Folstein MF, Folstein SE, McHugh PR 1975 "Mini mental state." A practical method for grading the cognitive state of patients for the clinician. J Psychiatr Res 12(3): 189–198.

Fraser RC 1982 Medical audit in general practice. Trainee 2: 142–145.

General Medical Council 2000 Confidentiality: Protecting and Providing Information. London: General Medical Council.

Greci LS, Kailasam M, Malkani S et al 2003 Utility of HbA(1c) levels for diabetes case finding in hospitalised patients with hyperglycaemia. Diabetes Care 26: 1064–1068.

Griffin SJ, Kinmonth A-L 1997 The management of diabetes by general practitioners and shared care. In: Pickup JC, Williams G (eds). Textbook of Diabetes, 2nd edn. Oxford, UK: Blackwell Scientific, Ch. 80.

Hippisley-Cox J, Yates J, Pringle M et al 2006 Sex inequalities in access to care for patients with diabetes in primary care. Br J Gen Pract 56: 342–348.

HMSO 1998 Data Protection Act 1998. Online: www.hmso.gov.uk/acts/acts1998/19980029.htm

Hutchinson A, McIntosh A, Feder G et al 2000 Clinical Guidelines for Type 2 Diabetes: prevention and management of foot problems. London: Royal College of General Practitioners.

Hutchinson A, McIntosh A, Peters J et al 2001 Clinical Guidelines for Type 2 Diabetes: diabetic retinopathy: early management and screening. Sheffield, UK: ScHARR, University of Sheffield. Online: http://www.shef.ac.uk/guidelines/

Hutchinson A, McIntosh A, Griffiths CJ et al 2002 Clinical Guidelines and Evidence Review for Type 2 Diabetes. Blood pressure management. Sheffield, UK: ScHARR, University of Sheffield. Online: http://shef.ac.uk/guidelines

Katz S, Ford AB, Moskowitz RW et al 1963 Studies of illness in the aged. The index of ADL: a standardized measure of biological and psychosocial function. JAMA 185: 914–919.

Khunti K 2006 Data presented at the Annual Professional Conference, Diabetes UK, Birmingham, UK, 30 March 2006.

Krans HMJ, Porta M, Keen H (eds) 1992 Diabetes Care and Research in Europe. The St Vincent Declaration action programme. Implementation document. Copenhagen, Denmark: World Health Organization, Regional Office for Europe.

Lee JD, Morrissey JR, Patel V for the Alphabet POEM Project (Practice Of Evidence-based Medicine) 2004 Recalculation of cardiovascular risk score as a surrogate marker of change of clinical care of diabetes people: the Alphabet POEM project (practice of evidence-based medicine). Curr Res Opin 20: 765–772.

Marshall SM, Flyvbjerg A 2006 Prevention and early detection of vascular complications of diabetes. BMJ 333: 475–480.

McIntosh A, Hutchinson A, Feder G et al 2002a Clinical guidelines and evidence review for type 2 diabetes. Lipids management. Sheffield, UK: ScHARR, University of Sheffield. Available online: http://shef.ac.uk/guidelines

McIntosh A, Hutchinson A, Home PD et al 2002b Clinical guidelines for type 2 diabetes: blood glucose management. Sheffield, UK: ScHARR, University of Sheffield. Available online: http://www.shef.ac.uk/guidelines/

McIntosh A, Hutchinson A, Marshall S et al 2002c Clinical guidelines and evidence review for type 2 diabetes: renal disease: prevention and early management. Sheffield, UK: ScHARR, University of Sheffield. Available online: http://www.shef.ac.uk/guidelines/

McIntosh A, Peters J, Young R et al 2003 Prevention and management of foot problems in type 2 diabetes: clinical guidelines and evidence. Sheffield, UK: University of Sheffield.

Meadows K, Abrams S, Sandback A 2000 Adaptation of the Diabetes Health Profile (DHP-1) for use with patients with type 2 diabetes mellitus: psychometric evaluation and cross-cultural comparison. Diabet Med 17: 572–580.

National Centre for Health Outcomes Development 2006 University of Oxford. Instrument for Diabetes: a Review. Available online: http://phi.uhce.ox.ac.uk/Final_diabetes_rvw_summ.pdf#8 (Accessed 7 May 2006).

National Diabetes Support Team 2006a Factsheet No. 14. Diabetes and the Healthcare Commission, March 2006. Available online: http://www.diabetes.nhs.uk/downloads/Factsheet_healthcare_commission.pdf (Accessed 9 May 2006).

National Diabetes Support Team 2006b Factsheet No. 15. Quality and Outcomes Framework Factsheet, January 2006. Available online: http://www.diabetes.nhs.uk/downloads/Factsheet_QOF.pdf (Accessed 10 May 2006).

National Diabetes Support Team 2006c Factsheet No. 16. Primary Care Commissioning Factsheet, March 2006. Available online: http://www.diabetes.nhs.uk/downloads/Factsheet_PBC.pdf

NHS Executive 1998 Information for Health. An information strategy for the modern NHS 1998–2005: a national strategy for local implementation. London: Department of Health. 1998. Available online: http://www.dh.gov.uk/assetRoot/04/01/44/69/04014469.pdf

NHS Information Authority Available online: http://www.connectingforhealth.nhs.uk/terminology/readcodes/index_html (Accessed 8 February 2007).

NICE Guideline Development Group and Recommendations Panel 2002a Inherited Clinical Guideline E. Management of type 2 diabetes: retinopathy – screening and early management. London: NHS National Institute for Clinical Excellence. Available online: http://www.nice.org.uk

NICE Guideline Development Group and Recommendations Panel 2002b Inherited Clinical Guideline F. Management of type 2 diabetes: renal disease – prevention and early management. London: NHS National Institute for Clinical Excellence. Available online: http://www.nice.org.uk

NICE Guideline Development Group and Recommendations Panel 2002c Inherited Clinical Guideline G. Management of type 2 diabetes: management of blood glucose. London: NHS National Institute for Clinical Excellence. Available online: http://www.nice.org.uk

NICE Commission for Health Improvement 2002 Royal College of Nursing, University of Leicester. Principles for Best Practice in Clinical Audit. Oxford, UK: Radcliffe Medical Press, March 2002. Available online: http://www.nice.org.uk

NICE, Diabetes UK and the NHS Executive Northwest 2002 Quality Indicators for Diabetes Services (QUIDS). Final Report of a Development Project Commissioned by NICE, Diabetes UK and the NHS Executive Northwest. Available online: http://www.quids.org.uk/

NICE 2006a Management of Hypertension in adults in primary care. NICE Clinical Guideline 34. London: NHS National Institute for Clinical Excellence. Available online: http://www.nice.org.uk/page.aspx?ozCGO34fullguideline

NICE 2006b Statins for the prevention of cardiovascular events: technology appraisal 94. London: NHS National Institute for Clinical Excellence. Available online: http://www.nice.org.uk/TA094

North of England Hypertension Guideline Development Group 2004 Evidence-based Clinical Practice Guideline: essential hypertension: managing adults in primary care. London: HMSO National Institute of Clinical Excellence.

Olivarus N de F, Beck-Nielsen H, Andreasen AH et al 2001 Randomised controlled trial of structured personal care of type 2 diabetes mellitus. BMJ 323: 970–975.

Renders CM, Valk GD, Griffin SJ et al 2001 Interventions to improve the management of diabetes mellitus in primary care, outpatient and community settings. Cochrane Database Systematic Reviews 1: CD001481.

Scottish Intercollegiate Guidelines Network 2001 Clinical Guidelines: management of diabetes. Edinburgh: Scottish Intercollegiate Guidelines Network (reviewed 2005). Available online: http://www.sign.ac.uk/guidelines/fulltext/55/index.html

Sinclair A, Cromme PVM, Rodriguez-Manas L et al 2004 Clinical Guidelines for Type 2 Diabetes. European Diabetes Working Party for Older People. Available online: http://www.eugms.org/academic/guidelines.jsp (Accessed 8 May 2006).

Tattersall R, Page S 1998 Managing diabetes in residential and nursing homes. BMJ 316: 89.

West Midlands Local Medical Committee. Available online: http://www.wmrlmc.co.uk/gms2/informationtechnology.htm#v8.0_20

WHO/IDF 1990 Diabetes care and research in Europe: the St Vincent's Declaration. Diabet Med 7: 360.

Williams B, Poulter NR, Brown MJ et al 2004 Guidelines for management of hypertension: report of the fourth working party of the British Hypertension Society, 2004. BHS IV. J Hum Hypertension 18: 139–185.

Wood D, Wray R, Poulter N et al 2005 JBS 2: Joint British Societies' guidelines on prevention of cardiovascular disease in clinical practice. Heart 91(Suppl. 5): 1–52.

APPENDIX 4

REFERENCES

Altman DG, Schulz KF, Moher D et al 2001 CONSORT GROUP (Consolidated Standards of Reporting Trials). The revised CONSORT statement for reporting randomized trials: explanation and elaboration. Ann Inter Med 134(8): 663–694 (17 April).